Analysing Community Work

Analysing Community Work

Theory and practice
Second edition

Keith Popple

 Open University Press

Open University Press
McGraw-Hill Education
McGraw-Hill House
Shoppenhangers Road
Maidenhead
Berkshire
England
SL6 2QL

email: enquiries@openup.co.uk
world wide web: www.openup.co.uk

and Two Penn Plaza, New York, NY 10121–2289, USA

First published 1995
First published in this second edition 2015

A catalogue record of this book is available from the British Library

ISBN-13: 978-0-335-24511-6
ISBN-10: 0-335-24511-0
eISBN: 978-0-335-24512-3

Library of Congress Cataloging-in-Publication Data
CIP data applied for

Typeset by RefineCatch Limited, Bungay, Suffolk

Fictitious names of companies, products, people, characters and/or data that may be
used herein (in case studies or in examples) are not intended to represent any real
individual, company, product or event.

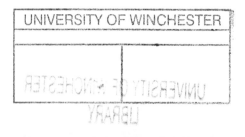

Praise for this book

"*Analysing Community Work provided a key text, tackling issues of theory and practice in accessible ways for some two decades. This second edition builds upon the strengths of the first, updating the book to take account of the major changes that have been taking place since then, both in Britain and internationally. Popple's critical consideration of the impacts of globalization, neo-liberalism, changing technologies, increasing inequalities and increasing concerns with environmental issues will be particularly welcomed. This edition will be essential reading for those who read and appreciated the first as well as for a new generation of readers.*"

Marjorie Mayo, Emeritus Professor of community development,
Goldsmiths, University of London, UK

"*Popple's book was one of the key overviews of British community work when it first appeared in 1995. In the last few years, the need for a revised and updated version has been increasingly obvious and Popple has now obliged. The last twenty years have seen substantial changes in the political, economic and organizational context within which community work operates and Popple has fully reflected this whilst remaining clear about its basic tenets and goals. This is a highly welcome addition to contemporary community work literature.*"

Gary Craig, Professor of Community Development and Social Justice,
Durham University, UK

For my son Daniel and in fond memory of my parents Ken and Sylvia

Knowledge begins with practice, and theoretical knowledge, which is acquired through practice, must then return to practice.

Mao Tse Tung

Contents

Acknowledgements

The second edition of *Analysing Community Work* has been a long time coming. Aware for some time that I needed to write a second edition, I always thought I would do it 'next year' when I would have a little more space and time. However, that time and space did not arrive and so other than make helpful notes, the project was delayed. Then, in the latter part of 2013, it became increasingly clear that there was a need to urgently produce a second edition. It was obvious the world had changed so much since the publication of the first edition in 1995 that it required an up-to-date analysis and comment alongside an informed commentary on the changes and possible future direction of community work. It was then that writing began in earnest. Now that task is complete, I would like to thank and acknowledge a number of people who helped me deliver this edition.

First, I would like to warmly thank the staff in the Department of Social Work at Hong Kong Baptist University and in particular Professor Tat-nam Petrus Ng, Dr Kwok-kin Fung and Dr Suet-lin Shirley Hung who facilitated my residence in the Department as a University Fellow for two stimulating months in early 2014 and who provided me with the space, resources and intellectual motivation to make substantial inroads into writing the book. They also restored my faith in what a university department should be with its emphasis on scholarship, critical thinking and quality liberal higher education.

Second, I would like to acknowledge and thank my supportive family and friends who have lived with me talking about and planning this book for some time. In particular, I would like to thank those who spent time with me in the UK during August 2014 in both rural Suffolk, and the New Forest and then in September of that year in the Algarve, Portugal offering me valuable feedback as I completed my writing. They gave me encouragement in my task and I am sure will be pleased it is now finished and published.

Third, I extend thanks to the publishers' reviewers for their helpful feedback of my second edition proposal. Their ideas and comments proved especially valuable when I actually came to put fingers to computer keyboard to write the book. I would also like to thank everyone at the Open University Press who assisted in the production of the book from the idea stage to the finished text and showed great patience as I worked to complete the project.

Finally, I would like to express a big thank you to students, practitioners, fellow academics and the many others who over the years have wittingly and unwittingly contributed to my thinking about community work theory and practice and in turn have led me to write what you will read here. However, of course, responsibility for the content of this book rests with me alone.

1 Introduction

The first edition of *Analysing Community Work* was published in 1995, since when the terrain in which community work is practised has changed considerably. Major events and developments at the international, national and local levels have all impacted on the way we understand and interact in the world we now inhabit and in turn how we experience community and neighbourhood. However, since 1995, despite the significant societal changes and assaults on the principles and practice of community work, the activity has remained true to its roots in questioning and, where necessary, challenging the power of the powerful as well as offering an alternative vision for now and the future.

The focus of this second edition therefore is to consolidate and build upon the understandings that were presented in the first edition and to reflect on the major changes that have taken place since then in the economic, political, social and cultural fields and to consider them in relation to the development of theories and practice of community work both in the UK and internationally.

Although community work can be considered to be a narrow localized limited activity, it can at the same time have a major impact on those involved and on the neighbourhoods that people live in and on the diverse communities which make up our societies and nations. Furthermore, community work is practised in most countries in the world and there are established forums, including international peer-reviewed journals that bring practitioners, academics and policy-makers together to enhance global links and to increase the influence of community work as a force for positive change.

While the term community work is used in this text, it is acknowledged that it is a generic term and within it sits a number of forms of the activity, including community development, community action, community organizing, community education, community care and community economic development, all of which will be discussed in this edition. In our analysis of community work we will be drawing on sources dedicated specifically to the dissemination of community work as well as referring to disciplines that inform the theory and practice of the activity including economics, sociology, social policy, social and economic history, and political science.

Since the publication of the first edition, there have been five major factors that have fashioned and influenced all our lives. One has been the rapid development and extensive spread of globalization; another is the power and influence of neo-liberal economics and politics; the third is the increase in the impact of technology; fourth is the increase in economic inequality both nationally and internationally; and the fifth is the influence of environmental politics and the advocacy of a sustainable future. These five interlinked factors are related to, and in the case of environmental politics a reaction to, the increasing control and pressure from enormous and powerful transnational corporations that have shaped the nature and influence of international trading while increasing economic and social inequality in and between countries.

The role of governments in this new world has also changed as they are now presently less interventionist in the delivery of welfare than during the period from after the Second World War to the early 1980s when the provision of state services in education, health, housing, social services and welfare almost everywhere was the mainstay of government spending. Instead governments in the twenty-first century are more focused on encouraging and supporting the market, including overseeing the transition of public bodies and functions to the private sector. The broad 'welfare consensus' of the latter half of the twentieth century has been replaced by a new political landscape that prioritizes 'residual welfare' approaches that embrace the notion of the mixed economy of welfare. 'Residual welfare' here is welfare that is provided at the minimal level, often for a temporary period, usually where there is clear evidence of need. As we will observe, these major changes and developments have had a profound effect on all our lives and the communities and neighbourhoods of which we are members. In fact, globalization and neo-liberalism have changed the type and extended the number of communities that now exist.

This edition will also consider the impact of new managerialism or New Public Management (NPM) on public services and community work. NPM is the thinking and practice of control of people and services that was largely developed in the private sector, and which is now being deployed in the public services. This logical positive approach to management, which is a cornerstone of neo-liberalism, emphasizes a hierarchical power structure and a model of working that can be used as a one-size-fits-all management method across any group or organization and is focused on defining and measuring specific outcomes. This often aggressive management style is used to monitor and regulate state-funded community work as it is deployed to dissipate neighbourhood anger and frustration. In particular, NPM is concerned with managing risk. As Beck (2008) argues, the loss of old certainties has led to unpredictable outcomes that society wants contained.

Globalization

Globalization is an often contested concept that has been with us for some time. In fact, the concept, if not the word, has been in existence since what we might now consider to be small-scale international trading of the first sea-faring civilizations. Nowadays, however, both small and large regional economies have become increasingly integrated through communication, trade and transportation. This has been described in the following manner:

> The flow of capital, labour, and technology has made all parts of the world more linked and, to different degrees, dependent on each other. Transnational corporations, such as Coca-Cola, Colgate-Palmolive, General Motors, Mitsubishi, Wal-Mart, Volkswagen, and large financial organisations and banks, for example HSBC, which produce or market services in more than one country, have played a major part in this development. Held et al. (1999) have estimated that transnational corporations account for two-thirds of all world trade and, according to Fortune (2006), 500 of these corporations had revenue much larger than most countries. For example, Exxon Mobil collected more revenue in 2005–2006 than individual major countries like South Africa, Saudi Arabia, Norway, and Turkey.
>
> (Popple 2012: 282)

Neo-liberalism

Neo-liberal economics and politics have at their core the view that the market is the best arbiter in the creation of wealth and distribution of income. The neo-liberal view is that the state is an impediment to the creation of wealth and at all costs should be reduced to a minimum. Keynesian economics, which was the main economic doctrine of Western countries in the period immediately after the Second World War, argues that investment in the state increases and sustains economic activity by developing and improving education and health and standards. However, the neo-liberal economic doctrine claims that, where possible, it is up to individuals to purchase their own education, health and social care, and so lessen their reliance on the state to provide these key services. This, it is argued, encourages private investment in these sectors, increases employment opportunities and produces profit for further development.

Increasing influence of technology

Technology has now permeated nearly every aspect of our daily lives with little sign that the rapid increase of the past twenty years will slow down. With the watch words of convenience, efficiency and speed much to the forefront, it is argued by many that these developments have brought us 'progress' both in our employment and in our homes. For example, as well as making our home lives more comfortable, technology has brought us diverse non-stop entertainment and communication which has allowed us to access and connect to people globally. This global communication is proving valuable at helping us to become more aware of events affecting people on the other side of the world as well as affecting the lives of those living closer to home.

Technology is also rapidly developing. For example, the mobile or cell phone which was first launched in 1973 solely for calling and messaging has now become a vehicle for a multitude of purposes, including playing games, watching movies, accessing social media sites, reading newspapers, magazines and books, and taking photos, now calling and messaging are a minority use. The question that is raised now is whether people are living in a virtual world of texting and social media sites and whether our lives have been devalued or lessened compared to before this technology was introduced. Has the introduction of many virtual relationships lessened our ability to create and enjoy meaningful relationships? Has this affected the way we interact in our various communities? Has the new technology produced new communities that are more meaningful than the traditional communities that had existed previously? Has technology prevented people from effectively talking to those they live with? Has the introduction of Facebook, Twitter and email provided us with forms of communication that are more exciting than sitting down with friends and family to undertake purposeful face-to-face communication? Is technology improving the quality of our lives while reducing our ability to have meaningful relationships with others? Or has technology helped us to extend our contacts and relationships while protecting and maintaining communication with those closest to us?

Increasing economic inequality

In 2014, the development charity Oxfam published two reports that reveal the growing economic inequality, both internationally and in the UK.

The first of these reports, *Working for the Few* (Oxfam 2014a) demonstrates that economic inequality is increasing at a rapid rate in the majority of countries, with seven out of 10 people living in countries where economic inequality has increased in the past 30 years. Arguing that the wealth of the world is divided in two, with nearly 50 per cent found in the richest 1 per cent and the remaining half among the remaining 99 per cent of the world's population, the report claims that the increasing inequality is impacting on global security and social stability. The report makes the point that the bottom half of the world's population owns the same as the richest 85 people in the world and continues:

> Some economic inequality is essential to drive growth and progress, rewarding those with talent, hard earned skills, and the ambition to innovate and take entrepreneurial risks. However, the extreme levels of wealth concentration occurring today threaten to exclude hundreds of millions of people from realizing the benefits of their talents and hard work.
>
> (Oxfam 2014a: 2)

Two months later, Oxfam produced a policy paper, *A Tale of Two Britains* (Oxfam 2014b), in which they state that the richest five families in Britain are wealthier than the bottom 20 per cent of the population. To quote the paper:

> Growing numbers of Britons are turning to charity-run foodbanks, yet at the same time the highest paid earners in the UK have had the biggest tax cuts of any country in the world. And whilst the low-paid workers are seeing their wages stagnate, the super-rich are seeing their pay and bonuses spiral up.
>
> (Oxfam 2014b: 1)

In the same year, the *Sunday Times* published its annual Rich List, which revealed that the 1,000 richest men and women in the UK had seen their wealth rise by 15.4 per cent of the previous year's total of £449 billion. Philip Beresford, who has compiled the Rich List since 1989, is quoted in the *Sunday Times* of 18 May 2014 as saying: 'I've never seen such a phenomenal rise in personal wealth as the growth in the fortunes of Britain's 1,000 richest people over the last year.'

Environmental politics and a sustainable future

In recent years science has made significant progress in assisting us to understand global warming and climate change and the impact this is likely to have on our societies in the coming years. The scientific consensus is that the Earth is warming up due to human action and climate change is now one of the greatest threats facing the planet, humans and animals.

For a number of years, transnational corporations, governments and several senior politicians have resisted the arguments and refused to deal effectively with climate change, arguing that regulation will do little to address what they claimed was unnecessary panic. This fitted well with the neo-liberal view of not intervening in matters of the market. However, in more recent times, we have seen the discourse shift and now an increasing number of corporations are arguing that climate change is likely to damage their profitability and they are wanting governments to act accordingly by significantly reducing greenhouse emissions and encouraging energy-efficient means of transport and the heating and air-conditioning of homes and workplaces, and to tackle polluted air, water and land.

While some corporations and governments are more inclined to tackle what some fear is a coming environmental catastrophe, however, there are still many who are engaged in the dangerous activity of fracking for shale gas, and opening up huge swathes of land and oceans for the drilling of oil and gas, while deforestation, water pollution, large-scale farming using chemicals, and the use of fossil fuels to produce energy go on unabated.

However, since the 1970s, environmental movements internationally have grown in influence and are bringing pressure to bear on governments and industry with the organization of product boycotts, highlighting the benefits of recycling and avoiding unnecessary packaging, encouraging less conspicuous lifestyles which focus on healthy living that involves eating less red meat, choosing more fresh foods that have been naturally grown and produced nearer to home, and reducing energy wastage and pollution by using, where possible, public transport, and choosing to walk and cycle. Many of these campaigns are locally based and deploy community work and, in particular, community action strategies, showing that environmental issues affect the daily lives of us all, from the air we breathe, the water we drink, the food we eat, and the transport and technology we use.

1995 and since

To contextualize the present situation outlined above, let us start by considering the political situation in the UK as it was when the first edition of *Analysing Community Work* was published in 1995 and when the Conservative Party were in government under the premiership of John Major.

Margaret Thatcher (1925–2013), who was the Prime Minister when the Conservatives were elected in 1979, was ousted by her Party as its leader in 1990 after concerns among her closest advisers and members of her Cabinet that she had politically misjudged the impact of the Poll Tax (the Community Charge), and had weakened her ministers' negotiating position in Europe. In the ensuing closely fought leadership election, she was replaced by the relatively unknown Cabinet minister, John Major.

Other than specific changes to the British National Health Service, the introduction of the National Curriculum in state sector schools, and the

increasing move to the mixed economy of welfare, the Conservative administrations under both Thatcher and Major did not make significant moves to
reorganize or radically transform the welfare state. Instead the government
concentrated their efforts on attacking and reducing the power of certain
elements of the workforce and particular working-class communities by de-
industrializing large swathes of traditional and previously powerful and
critical parts of the British economy, in particular, steel-making and coal-
mining, both of which were highly unionized. As a counteraction to this, the
Conservative government encouraged private investment (usually with
publicly funded incentives) and developments in the service industries,
high-tech sectors of the economy, and the finance sector which the
Conservatives deregulated to increase the flow of money and power into the
City of London.

In 1997, the Conservatives called a general election which was vigorously contested by the Labour Party, which during the previous two years
had refocused and rebranded itself to become 'New Labour' to distinguish
itself from its traditional working-class origins and socialist ideals. 'New
Labour' set out to capture the ideals of an electorate who were disenchanted
with the failing and accident-prone Conservative government. One commentator described the last few years of the Conservative administration in this
apt statement:

> For British voters, the Major years were remembered as much for
> the sad, petty and lurid personal scandals that attended so many of
> his ministers, after he made an unwise speech remembered as a call
> for old style morality ... a series of adulteries exposed, children
> born out of wedlock, a sex death after a kinky stunt went wrong,
> rumours about Major's own affairs (truer than was realised, though
> the press had the wrong person) and then an inquiry into whether
> Parliament had been misled over the sale of arms to Iraq, were
> knitted together into a single pattern of misbehaviour, which got an
> old name, 'sleaze'.
>
> (Marr 2007: 507)

'New Labour' were elected to government by a landslide majority vote and
swiftly began by reforming the welfare state and increasing investment in a
number of public services, including education, social work services and the
health service, while maintaining and developing the neo-liberal economic
policies of the previous Conservative administration. The savvy incoming
revitalized 'New Labour' administration had quickly acknowledged the fast-
changing nature of the economic circumstances they inherited and the new
world they were entering. With the collapse of Soviet socialism, 'New Labour',
like governments throughout the developed world, had concluded that the

only game in town was globalization and neo-liberalism, and prioritized making the economy more competitive against fierce international operations by freeing up aspects of the public sector for investment and development by the private market. In this neo-liberal consensus, 'New Labour' moved from the Conservative New Right position that had attacked and to some extent ignored welfare, and instead adapted and reshaped social insurance and state benefits with the purpose of moving people from 'Welfare to Work'. These central concepts were part of what was described as the 'Third Way' of politics which embraced a blend of neo-liberalism and social democracy (Giddens 1998).

In Chapter 4 we will be considering in more detail the period of UK history from 1995 to the present day and its impact on the development on community work. However, for our purposes here, we can see that there has been a seismic change from 1995 to the present day in the economic, social and political make-up of the UK and other developed countries. Chapter 4 will also consider the significant impact of the world banking crisis of 2008–09 which in the UK resulted in a massive publicly funded bail-out implemented by 'New Labour', which in turn moved the Conservative-led Coalition government of 2010 to introduce 'austerity' measures to promise to eliminate public finance deficits by 2015 (a promise they admitted in the Chancellor of the Exchequer's Statement in December 2012 that they were unable to fulfil).

Alongside the rapid development of globalization and neo-liberalism internationally there have also been a growing anti-globalization movement and campaigns and groupings opposed to increasing wealth and income inequality, both globally and in the UK. We will be examining the impact of these developments and what this means for community work in various places in this book. There will also be a consideration of communities and groupings that have been created by way of social media. These sites and the means of communicating have had a significant impact on the way that people communicate and the way in which they understand the world around them.

As with the first edition of *Analysing Community Work* my commitment has been to produce a book which will increase knowledge about community work and to continue to sharpen community work's critical edge and to contribute to a more effective practice that is centred on the values of democracy and social and economic justice. At the same time we need to be aware that community work encompasses a wide area of activity, is informed by a range of theories and knowledge bases, as well as the hopes and dreams of the multitude of people engaged in the activity. There are an enormous number of community work projects in every city, region and country, such that it is impossible to do full justice to this exciting, creative and diverse activity. However, I very much hope there is something for everyone in this analysis of community work.

The structure of the book

Definitions of community are important to community work theory and practice because, as we will uncover in Chapter 2, these definitions indicate different theoretical positions which will be discussed throughout the book. In
Chapters 3 and 4 we will examine the historical and structural contexts in
which community work has developed and in which they now take place.
Hence, in Chapter 3, we examine the development of community work since
the early part of the last century up to the 1970s, and in Chapter 4 we consider
the period of the economic crisis during the mid-1970s to present-day
developments.

In Chapter 5 we reflect on a range of theories which have influenced
community work and in Chapter 6 we look at how the theoretical themes
developed in Chapter 5 together with other thinking can assist us to create a
more effective practice of community work. This is followed in Chapter 7
with a consideration of community work models. Chapter 8 presents a discussion on community work in practice which will cover values, skills, education
and training and management. While this edition of *Analysing Community
Work* emphasizes the international nature of the challenges facing the activity, in Chapter 9 we consider some of the global organizations and journals
that are working to report and discuss innovative practices and developing
theories before referring to community organizing internationally, global
citizen action, and finally take a look at a community work project in Hong
Kong. Chapter 10 provides a conclusion and summary of some of the key
arguments presented in the book and then considers future directions for the
activity.

As an addition and departure from the first edition, each chapter ends
with questions that can be used to help direct reflection on the issues raised. It
can also be used by those engaged in teaching community work to assist
students think through the implications of the material presented.

In summary, this new edition contains a number of the key features of the
1995 edition as well as providing a substantial and critical update. We will be
considering a series of important and emerging themes of the past 20 years
including the impact that neo-liberalism and globalization have had on local
communities and in turn the role community work can play in addressing this
phenomenon; the increasing global concern for the future of the planet and its
resources and the role of community work in this; the stripping away of states'
responsibilities for the health, well-being and education of its citizens and the
expectation that individuals and communities will engage in voluntary work
for services to replace those previously undertaken by government agencies;
and, finally, and new to this edition we will spend time examining the practice
of community work internationally.

And finally . . .

When writing this book acknowledgement has been made that the UK is constituted of four separate countries, England, Northern Ireland, Scotland and Wales, each with their own distinctive rich cultural and national histories and with different understandings of what is meant by community work. This book does not provide space to consider the four countries in detail so the reader is asked to recognize that at times some generalizing has been made which does not fully reflect the patterns and forms of practice that have emerged within these countries. However, this should not prevent the reader from being informed of the role that community work can play both in the UK and internationally.

2 What is community?

Before we can successfully consider the theory and practice of community work it is essential to examine the notion of community. There is much talk about community in everyday life, for example, people talk about community spirit, or the loss or decline of a sense of community. What we can discover from these discussions is that these notions are frequently value-laden and subjective, which adds further to the problem of describing and analysing what community actually means.

However, it is not my intention in this chapter to pursue another definition of community, rather I would like to highlight some differing understandings and commentaries that reflect this imprecision and contentiousness. We will discuss later in the book the idea of moving power and opportunities to people in local communities or neighbourhoods, which is a commitment of all the major political parties. While this can be criticized as a strategy to reduce government spending, it is also a way of combating the voting populations' concern that they have little or no control over managerialist bureaucracies in the private and public sectors and also to more actively involve people in their local communities and neighbourhoods. All this confirms that the notion of community is important to consider in any exploration of community work.

The difficulties of defining community

Defining what the notion of community means, however, has never been straightforward. In fact, it could be described as one of the most challenging of sociological concepts to analyse successfully. Nevertheless sociology has played an important role in trying to unravel the term and this is well documented with numerous attempts to formulate an agreed definition (Wilmott 1963; 1989; Pahl 1966; Stacey 1969; Thorns 1976; Clark 1983; Golding and Sills 1983; Cornwell 1984; Wilmott and Thomas 1984; Fraser 1987; Black 1988;

Somerville 2011). More than 40 years ago, Bell and Newby (1971) found 98 different definitions of the term, while Abrams (1978: 11) declared that:

> The concept of community for its part is slowly being evicted from British sociology, not because there is agreement on the empirical collapse of community, but rather because the term has come to be used so variously and different relationships, identified as those of community, have been discovered in so many different contexts that the word itself has become almost devoid of precise meaning.

The nostalgic view of community

The nostalgic view of community is one which locates a 'golden age' of clearly defined and secure neighbourhoods in the historical period before the present one; sometimes colloquially called the 'good old days'. This is a recurring theme in British people's understanding of their own history, which is examined by Pearson (1983) in relation to street crime and hooliganism. The nostalgic view also represents community as a place of warmth, intimacy and social cohesion and this could be interpreted as a form of resistance and opposition to the significant changes that are taking place at the present time. The German sociologist, Ferdinand Tönnies has influenced the nostalgic view of community with his distinction between two kinds of social relationship (Tönnies 1955). One is based on affection, kinship, or membership of a community, such as a family or a group of friends. To describe this kind of relationship, Tönnies used the German word *Gemeinschaft*. The other kind of social relationship is based upon the division of labour and contractual relations between isolated individuals considering only their own self-interest. Tönnies referred to this society as *Gesellschaft*. Although Tönnies's terms need to be viewed as mental constructs, or ideal types, and do not correspond to any existing society, they do carry with it the suggestion that Western civilization is passing through the predominance of *Gemeinschaft* to a state of *Gesellschaft*. The implication is that many of the problems in contemporary society are due to this change. The term community in this paradigm contains associations which are often connected with security and nostalgic notions of how things were rather than how things are.

Community in 'soaps'

The media, in particular television and radio, uses the notion of community to great success in the popular programmes termed 'soaps'. Three long-running examples of television 'soaps' on British television are *Coronation*

Street, which portrays a northern urban working-class community, *Emmerdale*, which is set in a rural community in the Yorkshire Dales, and *EastEnders*, which provides viewers with a drama set in the fictional London East End postal area of Walford. This latter 'soap' features recognizable features of many neighbourhoods. For example, there are small businesses, including a convenience store, a pub, a fish and chip shop, a few streets and a square. 'Soaps' are regularly the most viewed programmes on terrestrial television in the UK, and the *The Archers*, a portrayal of the everyday lives of people living in a fictional rural village is the most listened programme on BBC Radio 4.

What is it about 'soaps' that make them so popular and what does it tell us about community? Geraghty (1991) argues that 'soaps' reflect the precarious nature of community. For instance, these fictional communities are often threatened by outsiders, such as developers or officious local authorities, or the plots present troublesome insiders such as bullies, petty criminals and gossips. According to Geraghty, one of the most important functions of British 'soaps' is to maintain the notion of community as a utopian ideal, particularly at a time when it is considered to be under threat. Geraghty believes that viewers and listeners can retreat into the 'soaps' world and leave national and international events behind. However, unlike what happens in real neighbourhoods, in the fictional dramas, real events are rarely discussed by the characters.

Nevertheless 'soaps' do present difficult, sensitive social and personal issues in accessible form. Issues such as HIV, teenage pregnancy, gay and lesbian relationships have been addressed as well as matters such as family secrets, racism, young people on the run, alcoholism, domestic violence and incest. Further, story lines have promoted education, including adult literacy, further and higher education, fathers reading bedtime stories to children, and teenagers studying for exams. It could be argued therefore that 'soaps' have provided an important educational role while offering entertainment, through the vehicle of modern-day morality stories.

With regard to community work it could be the argued that 'soaps' have damaged community life. Oral evidence from community workers indicates that the poor attendances at local residents meetings, the decrease in socializing outside the home, and a reduced engagement in community life can be attributed in part to the powerful draw of television and in particular the 'soaps'. Instead of engaging in their local neighbourhood, people are instead vicariously participating in an imaginary community in the comfort of their own home. We will consider the nature of home life in reducing people's participation in neighbourhoods a little later in this chapter.

Others argue, however, that soaps have brought people together, as people can discuss the latest developments in a 'soap' with their neighbours and others. Nonetheless the use of technical advances in the recording and watching and listening to programmes after they have been first broadcast means people can view them at leisure and therefore are no longer restricted from participating in community activities because they are watching a 'soap' at home at a specified time.

Romantic socialist views of community

Looking back historically, we can see that the concept of community was a central idea of Romantic socialists like the nineteenth-century textile designer, artist and writer, William Morris (1834–1896) (Thompson 1977; Meier 1978) and, from the same period, the art critic and patron, watercolourist and writer, John Ruskin (1819–1900) (Rosenberg 1961; Anthony 1983). In the twentieth century, the political theorist, economist and writer, G.D.H. Cole (1889–1959), who was primarily known for his libertarian socialist views, wrote about a decentralized form of government. He argued that there could be an active and participatory form of governing that was linked to people's workplaces and to the communities in which they lived (Cole 1918; 1920).

There have also been certain sections of the Labour Party that have advocated for socialism, based on the notion of community (Beilharz 1992). This view of community draws upon a nostalgic picture of working-class culture that is allegedly built on sound, deeply embedded socialist principles, which are waiting for the order to march behind the accredited leader of the day.

The nostalgic and the Romantic socialist concepts of community typify the problem of securing an agreed definition of community, although Williams (1976: 66) claims the term is rarely used disparagingly:

> Community can be the warmly persuasive word to describe an exist-
> ing set of relationships, or the warmly persuasive word to describe an
> alternative set of relationships. What is most important, perhaps, is
> that unlike all other terms of social organization (state, nation,
> society, etc.), it never seems to be used unfavourably, and never to be
> given any positive opposing or distinguishing term.

'Community' that is used to legitimate valued social achievement

Following on from the ideas of Raymond Williams, Webb (2011) has suggested that the notion of community is widely used to legitimate almost any valued social achievement. He argues that when the term is used in public discourse, it is a description or a reference to a range of normative aspects of social life, while placing these aspects in a favourable perspective. Community is therefore presented as a 'social ideal'. As Webb (2009) states in his earlier work, the term 'community' can be deployed to give a polish or spin to groups and organizations. This can be seen, for example, in the titles of state services: community schools, community police officers, community nurses, community mental health programmes, and so on.

Critics such as Cockburn (1977) claim that the term community hides the nature of powerful forces ranged against each other: the working class and the capitalist class. Cockburn states that the concept of community should highlight the reproduction of labour power that is mediated within communities: 'what we are involved in is struggle in the field of capitalistic reproduction' (1977: 163). Political and economic struggles, in her view, take place in the workplace, in schools, on the streets, and in families. Community workers can, according to Cockburn, emphasize that 'community' often means 'family' or more strictly 'women' (see also Wilson 1977). We shall be returning to the importance of women's role in the community and in community work at different places in the book.

Community as neighbourhood

Historically, for many people, community means neighbourhood with individuals understanding their lives in relation to the localities in which they reside. People know the boundaries of their community or neighbourhood, not by administrative boundaries but by what they consider to be the main constituents of the area. This is well described by Seabrook (1984: 2) when he states:

> [People] always know where their own neighbourhood ceases – at a main road, a canal, a row of shops, a park, a landmark. A neighbourhood is an area where the majority of people know by sight most of those who live there and probably recognize everyone of their own age group; know all the significant buildings and the central focus of the area – shops, schools, libraries, children's playgrounds, clinic, surgeries, youth clubs, Bingo halls, pubs, or whatever.

Seabrook's excellent analysis of the initiative by the local authority in Walsall, the West Midlands, to decentralize services in order that people in neighbourhoods could take greater control over the places in which they lived and worked also contains a sharp commentary on the assaults made on community life in working-class areas. He comments on what he terms as the 'sustained and untiring ideological assault on traditional working class values' (1984: 4) by the print media, who present a version of life in these communities as being a place where mugging and vandalism are frequent, while initiating and sustaining panics about 'child-molesters, drug addicts and alkies'.

The changing nature of community

Community and the UK's increasingly ethnically diverse population

Traditional views of community have often failed to fully recognize the ethnically diverse make-up of many neighbourhoods. Since the publication of the first edition of *Analysing Community Work* in 1995, England and Wales has become more ethnically diverse. However, the 2011 Census (ONS 2012) indicates that White remains the majority ethnic group with 48.2 million people (86 per cent of the population), and in this group White British was the largest group at 45.1 million (80.5 per cent) (this is the census tick box that is labelled as 'White English/Welsh/Scottish/Northern Irish/British'). Indian was the next largest ethnic group with 1.4 million people (2.5 per cent) followed by those indicating they are Pakistani and who comprise some 2 per cent of the population. The 2011 Census shows that London is the most ethnically diverse area, with the highest proportion of minority ethnic groups and the lowest proportion of the White ethnic group at 59.8 per cent. The next most diverse area with a White ethnic group at 79.2 per cent is the West Midlands.

Looking closer at the statistics for London, we see that it has above-average proportions of most minority ethnic groups, including African (7 per cent), Indian (6.6 per cent), and Caribbean (4.2 per cent). The capital also has the highest rate of Any Other White (these include those from other European countries, such as Polish people, the London-based French population, and those from South Africa, Australia, the USA, New Zealand, Canada and Russia) and who make up 12.6 per cent of the population residing there. London experienced the greatest proportional changes across the majority of the ethnic groups between the 2001 and 2011 Censuses with figures showing that in London, while the White British population decreased by 14.9 per cent, Any Other White and Any Other Asian populations had increased by 4.4 per cent and 3 per cent respectively during the 10-year period.

Moving away from the capital, we can see that Wales is the least diverse area, followed by south-west England and the north-west region of England. This data confirms that England and Wales remain countries where the predominant category of people are those who state they are White British, though there are regions, cities and neighbourhoods that reflect a good deal of diversity. For example, in Leicester, 28.3 per cent of the population are Indian, and Harrow in London has an Indian population that comprises 26.4 per cent of the local population. At the other end of the spectrum there is no record of an Indian population on the Isles of Scilly.

Rising individualism and declining social capital

We referred in Chapter 1 to the increasing impact of neo-liberal global capitalism on the contemporary world. The tentacles of this massive powerful drive has been felt by us all, no more so than in how we live in communities and neighbourhoods. The loosening of community ties, or arguably their reconfiguration, has in part been affected by the increasingly fast developments in information technology (IT) leading to new forms of online communication. These IT developments have both reflected and been fuelled by neo-liberalism. At the same time there has been an increase in geographical mobility and new forms of managing the public sphere. In the latter field we are witnessing the centralization of services, new managerialism, worker auditing and performance management.

One of the key aspects of the contemporary period is the recognition of rising individualism and declining social capital. The political scientist and professor of public policy Robert Putman found declining sources of social capital in the USA (Putman 2000). In this seminal work Putman argues that social capital, or social connections and knowledge that helps people to achieve their ambitions and goals, plays an important role for people in relation to their civic and community or neighbourhood life. Putman's conclusion

> was based on his finding that, over the previous 25 years, attendance at club meetings had fallen by 58%, family dinners were down by 33%, and having friends visit at home had fallen by 45%. He cited a number of reasons for this diminished social contact, including the fact that women, who have traditionally actively engaged more in neighbourhood and community affairs than men, were more likely to be employed in the labour force than previously.
>
> (Popple 2012: 284)

However, Putman (2000) attributed the major decline in community and civic engagement to the impact of television, the result of which has led to people spending time alone or with others watching TV programmes rather than spending time engaged in activities in their local communities and neighbourhoods.

Putman's view has been challenged by Chambers (2006) and Kraut et al. (2006) who argue that new technologies have increased rather than reduced people's contact with each other. For example, it has been estimated that in 1992 global internet traffic amounted to 100 gb per day. Twenty years later in 2012, this traffic had grown to 12,000 gb per second (Arthur 2013). While the majority of this is business traffic, the popularity of Facebook, Twitter, and Google has revealed that young people in particular are relating to 'each other through social networking sites and in the process creating dynamic new communities' (Popple 2012: 284). Despite these developments, Putman (2000) and Etzioni (1995) and other commentators have argued that focused neighbourhood programmes can, alongside new technology, do much to maintain and increase community cohesion. This approach has been described as 'moral communitarianism' and has been used by governments to build people's capacity through local involvement (Gray 2010). A contemporary example of this in the UK is the Coalition Government's 'Big Society' programme, which in essence means 'more community self-reliance and less government services, more volunteering and local entrepreneurial activity to look after the poor and needy rather than increased government resources' (Popple 2012: 285).

We will be examining the role of community action or community activism, as it is sometimes referred to, as an aspect of community work in Chapter 7. In brief, it is a discourse through which marginalized groups or groups intent on raising local issues can attempt to achieve positive collective gains. A central aspect of this discourse centres on using the community's potential for promoting social solidarity and collective action and is concerned with social justice. Writers have pointed to the failure of communitarianism to address the needs of the most disadvantaged groups (Shaw 2004; Craig et al. 2011; Ledwith 2011). Instead community activists argue there is a need for a radical transformative action (Gray and Boddy 2010).

Conclusion

We can see that definitions of community are elusive, imprecise, contradictory and controversial. Community has both descriptive and evaluative meanings, and is as much an ideological construct as a description of a locality. The term not only exists in a geographical and material sense but also reflects people's thinking and feeling as to where they believe a community exists (Popple 2002). Thus, other than elucidating the concept through its examination, one operational definition may be that community exists in three broad categories, as presented by Wilmott (1989: 2). The first is defined in terms of locality or territory which is often known as neighbourhood; the second as a communality of interest or interest group such as the 'black' community, or the Indian community or the Jewish community; the third, a group composed of people sharing a common condition or problem, such as alcohol dependency or cancer, or a common bond such as working for the same employer. Although this is a useful categorization, community must remain an essentially contested and imprecise concept.

Nevertheless the definition of community is important to community work theory and practice because, as we will discover, it helps us locate it in relation to this theoretical position. For example, one perception of community work is that it takes place in a pluralist society (and therefore in pluralist communities) and upon the premise of heterogeneity and inter-group competition. An opposing view perceives community work as taking place within communities and in a society that is based upon conflict and on the premise of class structure, economic and social inequality, discrimination and powerlessness, all of which are played out in communities and neighbourhoods. These competing and key understandings of community work will be examined at different places in the book.

Questions

1 Which communities are you engaged with?
2 Which ones are geographically located?
3 Which ones are communities of interest?
4 Do you consider there has been a decline in community spirit in your neighbourhood or does it enjoy positive supportive relationships between residents?

---

3 British community work
Early advances to the mid-1970s

Introduction

The focus of *Analysing Community Work* is an examination of contemporary community work theory and practice. However, to understand the present situation, we need to consider the developments that have taken place since the activity's emergence at the height of the British Empire and which have contributed to the situation we now are in. As an enterprise, the development of British community work has always been closely influenced by, and reflected in, the wider social, political and economic trends (see, for example, Baldock 1977; Loney 1983; Waddington 1983; Craig et al. 2011). In this sense the contemporary period is no different from the past. What is important for our discussions is the way in which trends, or features, in community work history have an influence upon, or link into, present-day developments.

Community work in the UK emerged from two contradictory and distinct forces: benevolent paternalism, as reflected in the work of the British Colonial Office, and the settlement movement; and collective community action, such as the 1915 Glasgow rent strikes, the unemployed workers movement, the suffragettes' right to vote campaigns, and the colonial struggles for independence. We begin Chapter 3 by considering these early forces. We will then reflect on the growth of community work during the pre- and post-Second World War period, through the expansion of the 1960s up to the mid-1970s. In Chapter 4 we continue this exploration by examining the different developments of community work from the 1970s to the present day.

Community work in the colonial tradition

It is difficult to give a precise date for the commencement of a recognizable form of British community work. However, community work was an integral feature of British imperialism and dates from before the twentieth century. The discussion surrounding the application by the British Colonial Office and other imperial agencies of community work techniques in developing countries is well documented (Halpern 1963; Mayo 1975; Marsden and Oakley 1982; Kwo 1984; Dominelli 2006). The main purpose of this form of community work was the integration of colonial territories into the capitalist system and to the benefit of Britain's entrepreneurs and government. The technique involved incorporating the indigenous ruling class into the colonial hegemony by affording them particular status and privileges. In return, support was given to the colonial domination through the collection of taxes and the establishment of legal and educational systems based on that in Britain. Craig (1989: 4) claims that while the inhabitants of British colonies may have gained materially and educationally from community work, the context in which this occurred was political: 'gains were made for local people, not by them'. Community work was to continue in developing countries after the dismantling of colonialism by playing a key role in combating the spread of communism.

Colonialism in developing countries did not go unchallenged by its populations and there is considerable evidence of rebellions by slaves, and struggles for independence, in countries under British domination (Judd 1996). The traditions and solidarity established among indigenous people during colonialism, and the resultant anti-colonial struggles, created a class consciousness which was brought to Britain by immigrants and their children (Gilroy 1993; Hazekamp and Popple 1997). As we will discuss later, this strengthened and resourced collective action by those from the colonies who settled in Britain, particularly from the early 1950s.

British community work: the early days

Community work within Britain commenced at a later date than its colonial equivalent. Engels (1844) provides us with a valuable critical commentary on the economic and social conditions of English cities in the early and middle part of the nineteenth century when the material circumstances of the working class were severely impoverished and when their political will was subordinated to the demands of capital.

To contextualize the period, we find that towards the end of the Victorian era (1837–1901) the British social structure was notably changing with the retreat of the aristocracy, the ascendancy of the bourgeoisie and the emergence of a more defined and increasingly politically organized urban working class. The period was also marked by the state beginning to take a permanent role in the welfare of its citizens (Thane 1989: vii).

From the early 1870s, the British economy experienced for the first time severe competition from the developing economies in Western Europe, in particular from Germany, and from the United States. As a consequence, the newly established bourgeoisie, which had made its wealth from industry, banking and commerce, and much of it linked to British imperialist ventures, became uncertain of its future. Meanwhile members of the new urban working class, which had appeared until then to have passively accepted their subjugated position, were becoming aware of their potential power through collective action and in particular through the increasingly influential trade union movement and the New Unionism of 1889 onwards. The advance of socialist ideas and the growth of Fabianism from 1884, and the influence of the writings of Karl Marx and Friedrich Engels, also played a part in raising the consciousness of large numbers of the urban population. The radicalization of the labour movement, the need to secure the support of the new working-class voters (mainly better-off skilled men), together with their awareness of the increasing numbers of people living in poverty, led sections of the already alarmed bourgeoisie to question the extent to which *laissez-faire* economic doctrines could effectively deal with persistent and worsening social conditions.

The threat to Britain's superior trading position similarly moved the government of the time to examine collectivist solutions to its economic and social dilemmas. In response, the Conservative governments of the turn of the century, and then the 1906–14 Liberal government, implemented a number of social and educational reforms which were intended to head off class conflict, and to benefit the long-term interests of British capital by equipping its workforce to compete both militarily and economically with its foreign rivals (Gough 1979: 62). These early collectivist solutions still left considerable room for the work of numerous Victorian charities and self-help groups, including the influential and powerful Charity Organisation Society (COS), which was established in 1869.

The COS as an early form of social work and the emergence of an alternative understanding of the impact of poverty on communities

The COS attempted to prevent the overlap of endeavours between the myriad of charities that emerged at the time. It was committed to the rational application of charitable assistance to those it considered 'deserving'. In order to separate the 'undeserving' from the 'deserving' poor, families in need were visited by volunteers, usually women drawn from the upper middle classes, who undertook a series of structured casework visits. This paternalistic and fundamentally judgmental activity was the commencement of what later became known as social work. (For an account of the origins and development of the COS, see Mowatt 1961.)

One of the founders of the COS, Canon Samuel Barnett, the vicar of St Jude's in Whitechapel, East London, became increasingly dissatisfied with the organization's inability to address the need to improve the living and working conditions of the poor and argued that it was possible to establish settlement houses in poor neighbourhoods which could offer educational and recreational opportunities for those living in disadvantaged communities.

Following in the wake of the work of the British economic historian, Arnold Toynbee (1852–1883), who with his colleagues was committed to improving the living conditions of the poor, and who had spent their summer vacation of 1883 living in Whitechapel in order to study poverty, Barnett formed the University Settlement Association. Inspired by the ideas and work of Arnold Toynbee, Samuel Barnett and his wife Henrietta Barnett founded the first university settlement in 1884, a little after Toynbee's death. Located in Commercial Road, East London, the first settlement was named Toynbee Hall.

Toynbee Hall: the first British settlement

Toynbee Hall, which has been described as the 'Mother of Settlements' (Rimmer 1980), had as its philosophy a belief that if the poor were treated as having the same worth as the rich, class barriers would disappear, and material improvement would increase, and this was influential in the early development of community-based intervention in poor areas.

Among its student residents from 1903 to 1907 was William Beveridge, who later was the prominent reforming civil servant who advocated the introduction of universal welfare benefits and the welfare state, and Clement Atlee from 1909 to 1910, who became the leader of the British Labour Party from 1935 to 1955 and was Prime Minister from 1945 to 1951 (Harris 1977: 43). American students also stayed at Toynbee Hall, and in 1887 they started the College Settlement Association in the United States of America (Rimmer 1980: 2).

By the end of the nineteenth century 30 settlements based on the model of Toynbee Hall had been established in the UK, many in university towns and cities. The settlements were usually residential and university students (who were drawn from the upper and middle classes) were able to spend some of their free time living and working in poor neighbourhoods, offering a range of educational classes and welfare services (Thane 1989: 23).

Beginnings of community work in the settlement movement

We can see that the settlement movement contained within it the beginnings of British community work. It was part of a wider response to a range of social, economic and political difficulties facing neighbourhoods in Victorian and Edwardian Britain. Although community work within Britain was not used in the overt manner that it was in the colonies, its aim was not entirely dissimilar. Instead of the Colonial Office being the main channel for community activity, it was the Anglican Church and the universities that initiated projects, organizations and movements. The Church and the universities were powerful establishment institutions that played a strategic role in the growth of community work as a means of both dissolving dissent between the social classes in urban areas, and of addressing the issue of poverty in its broadest sense (Jones 1977). Like those involved in the COS, the community work innovators were upper- and middle-class reformers rather than state functionaries or even political revolutionaries. Many of them in fact reflected the 'reforming evangelical trend in the Church of England' (Parry and Parry 1979: 24).

The 1915 Glasgow tenants strike: an early form of community action

We have noted the increasing strength and confidence of the labour movement during the late nineteenth and early twentieth centuries. In response, the state, for reasons discussed above, introduced a number of reforms to advance the well-being of the working class and, in turn, the profitability of capitalism. The reforms were also aimed at integrating the working class into the values and ideals of the status quo in order to ensure the stability and security of the bourgeoisie. However, resistance to the dominant hegemony was found where class consciousness was strongest and where support could be drawn from 'regional and national loyalties, especially in the Celtic fringe' (Bedarida 1990: 134). It is not surprising to note, therefore, that one of the earliest recorded forms of community action was in the city of Glasgow where thousands of tenants were involved in a rent strike, with strikes and protests spreading to other cities and towns with calls for lower rents and improved housing (Darner 1980). Clydeside employers supported the workers' struggle because the higher rents were creating an unsettled workforce and deterring labour from moving to the area. The outcome was the Rent and Mortgage Interest (Rent Restriction) Act 1915, which restricted rent and mortgage interest rates (Melling 1980).

Working-class collective action was also prevalent in the 1920s and 1930s with the growth of the National Unemployed Workers' Movement (Hannington 1967; 1977). Craig (1989: 4) believes this development was the first attempt to link struggles in the home with those in the workplace. There is some evidence to support this, though Bagguley (1991: 108) reveals that women were marginalized by the dominance of men in organization of the Movement.

The increasing recognition of women's role in community

The suffragette movement also played a part in the growth of collective action, though in this case it was almost exclusively bourgeois (Rowbotham

1977; 1992). The direct action and often illegal tactics – including delegations, public demonstrations, and interruption of meetings, and then hunger strikes – were aimed at raising public consciousness for female suffrage. However, it was not until after women had been given new roles in the First World War that they were able to achieve the franchise in 1918. While the 1918 Representation of the People's Act gave the vote to women over 30, it was not until 1928 that women gained voting equality with men.

The inter-war period: the emphasis on community integration to counter worker unrest

While the British economy was in a depressed state during the inter-war period, there were a number of innovations in the community work field, including the establishment by Henry Morris in 1928 of the first Cambridgeshire village college. This innovative, comprehensive community provision marked the commencement nationally of the gradual and often slow advance of community schools and colleges (Ree 1973; McCloy 2013).

Another important innovation that was to have an impact on the growth and direction of community work was the establishment of community centres that were funded by the government and the voluntary sector. This intervention was in response to growing unemployment and the public concern for the settling of newcomers in new council estates. This initiative was intended in part to counter the alternative facilities offered by the National Unemployed Workers' Movement, whose centres were considered by the National Council for Social Service as potential threats to 'national stability' (Hanson 1972: 636).

We can see that the development of community work during the economically depressed inter-war years was largely instigated by government-supported agencies, and by the increasingly significant settlement movement. These developments were primarily aimed at integrating into broader society those communities suffering from the effects of severe unemployment and undergoing a period of unsettling physical transition.

Worker unrest, the growth of mutual aid organizations, and a divided Britain

On the industrial and political front there was a great deal of worker unrest during the 1920s which culminated in the General Strike of 1926. According to Beatrice Webb's diaries this was to prove to be 'one of the most significant landmarks in the history of the British working class' (quoted in Cole 1956: 92).

The ideology of self-help, which was a feature of the Victorian middle class, was also an aspect of working-class life at this time, with the development of the co-operative movement, adult education (the Workers' Educational Association was established in 1903), friendly societies as well as trade unionism all reflecting an 'ameliorative rather than revolutionary social philosophy' (Fraser 1984: 108). Nevertheless, as Payne (2005: 34) observes, 'Mutual help became allied to efforts at social reform with broad application for the benefit of working people, rather than systems of individualized personal help.'

Britain in the late 1930s was a divided country. Those in work were enjoying rising real incomes and living standards, while those who were unemployed were experiencing increasing poverty (Stevenson and Cook 1977). It is difficult to trace the development of community work from this period until the end of the Second World War, though we do know that a wide range of voluntary bodies, including the Citizens' Advice Bureau (formed in 1939) and the Women's Royal Voluntary Service (which was formed in 1938 and now called the Royal Voluntary Service), were to play a part in the war effort (Calder 1971).

Wartime Britain: a sense of national solidarity and demand for change in civil society

By the early 1940s, in the Second World War, the threat of the invasion of Britain by Nazi Germany had an increasing impact upon the British people. After three decades of bitter class confrontation, there was a growing consensus, coupled with a clearer sense of national solidarity, all aimed at defeating the common enemy, Nazi Germany, led by Adolf Hitler. Writing about the English, one of the leading historians of the time, A.J.P. Taylor, describes this as 'a brief period in which the English people felt they belonged to a truly democratic community' (Taylor 1965: 550). This experience of solidarity led Richard Titmus to comment that there was after the war a new attitude towards social policy, with general agreement and willingness 'to accept a great increasing of egalitarian policies and collective state intervention' (quoted in Harris 1981: 43). This was to lead to the post-war social-democratic consensus and an organized and extensive welfare state.

Community work in social democracy

Post-war austerity but growing national confidence

The early post-war years in Britain were a period of social reform premised on a harmony of mutual interests between capital and labour, an agreement which became known as the social-democratic consensus. The agreement was built on the labour movement's demand that the gains from the capitalist system should be shared with working people. In return, the ruling elite accepted that it could, and should, provide improvements to working-class life and conditions. This is a central and enduring concept in the developing relationship between the state and the British people and from which modern community work emerged.

The British public's wish to see a political consensus was demonstrated in the overwhelming victory of the Labour Party in the 1945 General Election. The Labour Party, with a manifesto arguing for higher and more proportional direct taxation in return for greater state provision, gained a substantial, 146-seat majority with 47.8 per cent of the votes cast (Butler and Sloman 1976). This gave Labour a mandate to carry out sweeping economic changes, structural social reforms and to introduce the modern welfare state.

The British economy and indeed the international economy prospered from a long economic boom, which stretched from the mid-1940s until the late 1960s and early 1970s, and was reflected in rising levels of output and living standards, low unemployment, and expanded trade (Harris 1988: 14). For those in employment there were improvements in their working conditions together with the benefits of longer paid holidays. It was also a period when a complacent air of the affluent society pervaded institutions, while conventional wisdom held that the economy was benefiting everyone. This was further reflected and encouraged by government ministers (Bogdanor and Skidelsky 1970; Sked and Cook 1984). Meanwhile community work played a part in the acceptance of the social-democratic consensus with the continuing activity through local councils of social services and the community centres in new housing estates. Thus, the dominant mode of community work was largely within the voluntary sector (Thomas 1983: 18) and reflected the tradition of benevolent paternalism.

The official recognition of poverty and the changing nature of community life

The prevailing and fundamentally complacent view that the British economy was delivering the affluent society to all its citizens was being challenged by the late 1950s. One challenge emerged with the growth of sociology and social policy as critical social science subjects and led, in part, to the rediscovery and recognition in the 1960s of poverty in many areas of the UK (Abel-Smith and Townsend 1965; Hobsbawm 1968; Coates and Silburn 1970). At the same time a number of community studies were being carried out that revealed the decline of traditional (and often idealized) working-class spirit, and working-class communities, and the breakdown of social control (Loudon 1961; Wilmott 1963; Frankenberg 1969). At the grassroots level there were examples of community action, most notably in the form of squatting in government-owned premises, because of the shortage of adequate housing provision by the state (Craig 1989: 6). The mass slum clearance and the creation of new towns of this time were to further raise concerns about the break-up of communities and the impact on individuals and families (Heraud 1975).

The emergence of community work theory

From the early 1950s, community work theory, which was beginning to be developed in North America, began to have an impact upon theory and practice in Britain. Perhaps the most influential book on community work of the time was written by a Canadian, Murray Ross (1955). Smith (1979: 65) states that the work of Ross 'captured the imagination of staff in councils of social service because it suggested there was a theoretical basis for their work, and set about community work as neighbourhood work . . . and . . . as interagency work'. So while community work practice was emerging in Britain, it was in North America that community work theory began to surface. These early texts were then used by British community workers.

The first British attempts to construct a distinct theory of community development can be seen in the writings of T.R (Reg) Batten, who had been engaged in British agency-funded community work in Nigeria from 1927 to 1949. Batten was critical of the use of community work as a means to perpetuate colonial domination (Batten 1967: v). During this time he became associated with the non-directive approach to community work which, as we will note later was to influence early community work training (Batten 1957; 1962; 1965). For an excellent account of the life and work of Batten, see Lovell (2009).

The Younghusband and Calouste Gulbenkian reports

In Britain, the influential report by Younghusband (1959) identified community work as a third method of social work intervention alongside case work and group work. The work by Kuenstler (1961) was to develop this concept, and by the beginning of the 1960s there were a number of workers who described themselves as 'community workers', and the term 'community work' was in general use (Jones 1983: 1). By the middle of the decade, community work was 'tied intellectually to social work' (Thomas 1983: 21), though it was not till later in the 1970s that it was possible to identify the practice within social services departments.

The advance of British community work was gathering pace when the Calouste Gulbenkian Foundation (1968) published a significant report which was to promote and debate the nature and purpose of the activity, while exploring the role of community workers and the issues they confronted. Jones (1983: 2) believes the lack of attention in the report to the conflictual relationship between community work and political activity did not reflect the extensive discussions within the working party, which was drawn from practitioners. One can only speculate as to the reasons for this. Perhaps one reason for the final consensus was due to the influence of its chairperson, Dame Eileen Younghusband, who perceived community work as a new form of social work (Thomas 1983: 30). Another reason may have been the power of the prestigious and wealthy Gulbenkian Foundation which funded the report. What we know is that the report of the Seebohm Committee (HMSO 1968) was to have similar significance in the development of the activity by confirming the adoption of community work methods by social work and in helping to create the occupation of community work.

The influence of Saul Alinsky

It is worth pausing here a moment to note the work of Saul Alinsky (1909–72) who is considered by many to be the founder of community organizing. Alinsky, who was born in Chicago and studied at the University of Chicago, had witnessed and examined the impact of deprivation and poverty on many of the city's population, especially during the US Depression of the 1930s. The experience was to politicize him and he believed he could play a part in improving the living conditions of people (mainly African-Americans) living in the ghettos of a number of American cities. Alinsky was to prove to be a charismatic and influential coordinator and leader whose methods led to the building of powerful organizations that challenged the 'politically and economically powerful organizations that were oppressing people within the community' (Beck and Purcell 2013: 2). One of the keys to Alinsky's success was to recognize that people are primarily motivated by self-interest. However, as Beck and Purcell (2013: 7) argue:

> This is not to say that community organizing is an individualized practice. On the contrary, it recognizes that the wellbeing of individuals is interwoven with that of others. This viewpoint is echoed in rational choice theory, which is based on the assumption that individuals maximize their self-interest. Since it is clear that an individual has limited potential to influence the wider world, it is rational and self-serving to create relationships and to support people who in turn will support you, thereby developing stocks of social capital that you can draw on in the future.

Although Alinsky's work was centred on American cities, his theories and practices have been adopted elsewhere, including the UK, where films of his work have been used in community work training. Importantly too is his famous text *Rules for Radicals* (Alinsky 1971) which presents readers with his central ideas and analysis and remains a classic text for those striving for greater social and political justice.

The rapid growth of British community work

From 1968 until the mid- to late 1970s community work grew as an activity in both statutory and voluntary sectors, as the state became increasingly involved in the task of addressing social, political and economic change.

This section begins by considering the national and international events that created a sense of change in the late 1960s. It continues by exploring two major influences on community work during this period: the Urban Programme and the National Community Development Projects. We then consider other important contemporary themes, including: extra-parliamentary activities; the work of the Gulbenkian Foundation; the influence of the women's movement; the concern with immigration and racial unrest; plans for developing inner-city areas; the role of the Manpower Services Commission; and the continuing decline in the British economy and the resultant industrial, political and social changes.

'The times, they are-a-changin'

The year 1968 proved to be a watershed in world-wide changes and challenges as well as a landmark in the evolution of community work. In the wider political context, 1968 was a year of revolt, rebellion and reaction throughout the world, with a catalogue of events that included: the student and worker struggles in Paris during May of that year; student demonstrations and occupations at universities in several countries, including Britain; the Vietnamese Tet Offensive against American imperialism; world-wide protest and demonstrations against US involvement in Vietnam; racial riots in the United States; the assassinations of the black American civil rights leader, Martin Luther King, Jr, and the American politician, Democratic Senator and civil rights activist, Robert Kennedy; the introduction of the US Civil Rights Bill; the invasion and occupation of Czechoslovakia by Warsaw Pact troops; civil rights activists in Derry, Northern Ireland, defying the government's ban on their marching; and the first mass open-air rock concert in Britain. It was a year of turmoil and change and, to quote one commentator: 'a year after which nothing could ever be the same again, a year which divides epochs, and a year which branded a generation for life' (Kettle 1988: 3).

By the late 1960s the British economy was experiencing a deepening economic crisis, with worsening unemployment, and a lack of international competiveness which led the Labour government to devalue the pound sterling and to deploy new forms of social intervention in those areas thought to be worse affected by the country's changing fortunes.

The government, aware of the need to respond to the growing economic and social changes, commissioned a number of reports; the conclusions of which can be read as a recognition that the welfare state had failed to meet the needs of disadvantaged and marginal groups, and that capital needed the continuation of a stable, well-integrated workforce. These reports advocated further intervention in working-class areas which was to assist in increasing the profile and value of community work.

- *The Ingleby Report* (Home Office 1960) recognized the role of family advice centres and the need to undertake preventive social work with children and young people, and led to the establishment of neighbourhood and family centres that helped boost the advance of community work as a valid form of intervention.
- *The Plowden Report* (DES 1967) also made a contribution to community-based interventions as it advocated a significant programme of positive discrimination in the primary education sector, including the development of local projects aimed at strengthening the relationship between the home, school and the community.
- *The Seebohm Report* (HMSO 1968), mentioned earlier, was a key document that advocated a role for community work, this time within social work service provision and confirmed the role of community as an important one in recognizing the value of locality.
- *The Skeffington Report* (HMSO 1969) recommended increased, if limited, public participation in planning and enabled community workers to engage with residents in neighbourhoods affected by proposed changes.
- *The Fairbairn-Milson Report* (DES 1969) encouraged youth workers and youth work managers to develop a community perspective and highlighted the impact community work could make in neighbourhoods.

Two major government innovations of long-term significance in the development of British community work that developed at the same period were the Urban Programme, established in 1968, and the National Community Development Projects, launched in 1969, as an element of the Urban Programme. These two significant developments are now considered.

The Urban Programme

The Urban Programme emerged as a response by the Labour Government to Enoch Powell's 'Rivers of blood' speech given in Birmingham in April 1968.

Powell, a Conservative Front Bencher, predicted the emergence of racial tension in British cities similar to that witnessed in the United States (Powell 1968: 99). Powell's inflammatory speech led to him being removed from his political position by Edward Heath, the Conservative Party leader. Nevertheless his views received widespread popular support, including among some dock workers, 1,000 of whom marched on the Houses of Parliament as a sign of solidarity and support for the former Shadow Defence Secretary.

The government, fearing that support for Powell's racist perspective would increase racial tension in the country, moved with speed and a month later had launched the Urban Programme which was designed to address social problems in those areas experiencing deprivation. The government's concern was to be seen to be acting on rising public panic to immigration and 'race' relations (Foot 1969: 112). With unemployment increasing from the early 1960s, both the Conservative and Labour Governments had begun restricting immigration from the developing world while at the same time attempting to enhance the integration of those immigrants already settled in the UK.

The Urban Programme was, therefore, part of a policy of containing the 'problem' of newly settled immigrants living in urban areas. It was not a coincidence that at central government level 'race' relations and the new Urban Programme were the responsibility of the same parliamentary under-secretary (Edwards and Batley 1978: 38–9).

The Urban Programme was not restricted to 'black areas' partly 'for fear of provoking accusations of favoured treatment for immigrants' (Loney 1983: 34), and it proved ineffective at reaching ethnic minority groups (Demuth 1977). In practice, many local authorities and voluntary organizations in different parts of Britain applied through the Urban Programme for aid to combat local pockets of deprivation, defined in terms of social indicators: unemployment, overcrowding, large families, poor environment, immigrant concentrations, and children in care or in need of care. In concert with the social-democratic consensus of targeting the funds to 'areas of deprivation', the state allowed no recognition of the 'widespread consequences of economic and industrial decline as they affected the working class in general' (Bolger et al. 1981: 122).

Through various Urban Programme initiatives millions of pounds were distributed to a plethora of community work projects and by 1987 it was supporting approximately 4,000 voluntary and community work projects (Taylor and Presley 1987) though by the same time Urban Programme resources were declining in real terms (Whitting et al. 1986).

In fact, funds allocated to the Urban Programme were 'dwarfed' by financial cuts applied to inner-city local authorities (Benyon and Solomos 1987: 193). However, the Urban Programme successfully continued for many years as it was focused on targeting relatively small amounts of money for signifi-cant but politically 'safe' activities and projects which were to receive warm appeal in the communities in which they were located, with provision for children and community projects being two areas that attracted regular funding over the years (Laurence and Hall 1981: 92–3).

The Urban Programme was also used by the Conservative Government during the 1980s to employ workers with the young unemployed and to support financially projects such as those targeted at young black offenders, community-based projects catering for 16–21-year-old unemployed people, and neighbourhood projects involved in a range of activities including youth work, play schemes and clubs for older people.

Overall, it can be argued that the Urban Programme greatly assisted British community work to grow and diversify and to stimulate the development of the activity in both the voluntary and statutory sectors. However, the pervasive feature of the various schemes was their use of short-term funding which did little to counter the reputation of community work as being experimental and tokenistic.

The National Community Development Project

The other major development of state-supported community work, launched in 1969, was the National Community Development Project (NCDP). Like the Urban Programme it was part of a wider initiative to address social disharmony at a neighbourhood level. It was also developed out of concerns voiced in many quarters that certain sections of the population were failing to successfully respond to the changing social and economic circumstances. Influenced and informed by the American 'War on Poverty' Programme, the NCPD was developed by the Home Office to improve the delivery of a range of social services and to co-ordinate already established community and local authority based projects. The 12 neighbourhood Community Development Projects (CDPs), which were funded by a combination of local and central government finance, had a brief to identify where other services could be introduced.

When launched, the projects supported a community pathology model of poverty that argued that people in disadvantaged communities failed to compete in the marketplace because of internal community or personal problems rather than because of structural inequalities. The projects were intended to assist people to use the social services more constructively and to reduce dependence on these services by stimulating community change (Mayo 1980). However, the workers and researchers employed on the local CDPs, which were situated in 'deprived areas' (Batley, Canning Town, Cumbria, Coventry, Glyncorrwg, Liverpool, Newcastle upon Tyne, North Shields, Oldham, Southwark and Paisley), rejected the predominantly Conservative explanations of poverty and inner-city deprivation, many of which were articulated by Keith Joseph, who was aligned to the 'cycle of deprivation' view of poverty in society (Joseph 1972). Instead, the CDP staff produced a radical critique that demonstrated the structural basis of poverty was perpetuated by capitalist relations and by social structures, and which created an unequal distribution of resources and power throughout society. The CDP staff argued that the poor inhabitants of the 'deprived areas' were considered to be essential for the continuance of capitalism. (Unfortunately space does not allow me to discuss the examples of the locally based CDPs. The Appendix provides a select bibliography of CDP reports and publications.)

Successive governments did not take kindly to the project teams' radical analysis and by 1976 central government had withdrawn its funding from what it had originally conceived as an experiment in the co-ordination of central and local government and voluntary sector resources (Green 1992). The central state was not the only critic of the CDPs; there is evidence that the team's Marxist analysis was also criticized by local authorities and communities for its radical perspective (McKay and Cox 1979). However, the point should not be lost that the CDPs' analysis (that structural inequalities were the root cause of poverty and an integral aspect of capitalism), was the central reason for the state's swift action to silence the radicals (Loney 1983). The NCDP proved to be the most controversial of all the government-sponsored community work programmes, and was also the clearest example of the radical and socialist approach to community work theory and practice. Overall it was one of the most important and defining initiatives in the evolution of British community development (see Popple 2013).

Further significant developments

By the end of the 1960s, there were a number of strands feeding into the development of community work. We have noted the impact of national and international world events which were to assist in the creation, particularly among young people, of a counter-culture and a new thinking and understanding of a challenge to the political, social and economic affairs of the period (Popple 2009). The Labour Party in office was to disappoint the social reformers who were hoping for a transformation in society and a move to a greater redistribution of Britain's wealth and income. The rise of the Campaign for Nuclear Disarmament as a vehicle for protest against the government pursuit of deploying nuclear weapons, and the development of single-issue pressure groups such as Shelter and the Child Poverty Action Group – which was set up at Toynbee Hall in 1965 (Briggs and Macartney 1984) – as a result of the rediscovery of poverty, were symptomatic of extra-parliamentary activities. These pressure groups were formed as a challenge to and in response to the disillusionment with conventional politics. These, together with the growing number of critical intellectuals in the social sciences, the radical ideas and literature of the emerging New Left, the decline of Britain's economic performance, the increasing concern in government circles that the welfare state was failing to integrate certain individuals and communities, and the fear of urban unrest focused primarily around the issue of immigration, led in different ways to an increase and expansion in locally based community work projects. As we have noted, the majority of these projects were initiated and funded by government, with community work being one of a number of interventions aimed in part at diffusing possible radical protest and managing economic and social change. There was, however, a profusion of locally initiated community action projects that centred on development concerns and rent increases. Similarly, the government-funded community programmes were, as we have seen in the example of the local CDPs, staffed by workers influenced by a political analysis that was critical of the structural inequalities within a capitalist society. However, as Waddington (1983: 42) recalls, the analysis of the majority of community workers 'basically reflected a gut reaction against bureaucracy and a rather unspecific idealism which owed rather more to the ideals of the "alternative society" than to the thinking of the New Left'.

Among other significant features of community work's evolution was the establishment in 1966 of the Association of Community Workers (ACW), which was an attempt to coalesce support for the practice of community work and to help provide a clearer identity for its practitioners. Another important development during the same year was the launch of the *Community Development Journal* (CDJ) by Oxford University Press. While the CDJ remains one of the leading journals in the field, the ACW has since been dissolved.

The CDJ emerged out of discussions among community development practitioners and educators returning from the British colonies. These included the above-mentioned Reg Batten, and Peter Du Sautoy, who was previously Director of Social Welfare and Community Development in Ghana, and who on his return to the UK in 1960 was appointed as a lecturer in Fundamental Education and Community Development at the University of Manchester. Du Sautoy, Batten and others wanted to bring to the UK the lessons learnt from the colonies that community development could successfully address the country's neighbourhood problems. With the support of Oxford University Press, the CDJ was launched with Du Sautoy as its first editor, with the aim of offering readers in the UK and elsewhere a developing community work literature (Popple 2008).

Although there is no reliable statistical data to provide a dependable indicator of the growth of community work during this period, it is agreed that by the early 1970s community work was rapidly developing and, to quote Waddington (1983: 42) further, was feeding off

> the annual surplus of a growing economy and was part of a system of
> public sector redistribution to disadvantaged and marginal groups, a
> form of 'kitty bargaining' which helped to give substance to the

claims of pluralist politics. The progressive adoption of community work by the state has – amongst other reasons – followed recognition of its value as a tool to reinforce a flagging belief in social democracy, especially amongst economically marginal groups.

During the 1970s the state continued to be the prime funder of community work, both through the public sector and in its grant aid to the voluntary sector. One of the most significant community work grant-making trusts outside the state was the Calouste Gulbenkian Foundation, who funded interventions that were experimental and innovatory. The Foundation was also to play a significant role in raising the profile of community work through its many publications, training events, conferences and national networking and was able to claim that it had a role in government policy-making in relation to community work and in the establishment of the Federation of Community Work Groups (Mills 1983: 86).

The increasing significance of gender and 'race'

The women's liberation movement re-emerged in Britain during the early 1970s after 'the stirrings of consciousness in the late 1960s' (Rowbotham 1989: xii) and the first women's liberation conference of 1970. This pivotal conference was to demand equal pay for women, equal education and employment opportunities, 24-hour nurseries, free contraception and abortion on demand. The conference, however, did not catch the public's imagination in the way that the 1968 strike by female sewing machinists at the Ford motor car plant at Dagenham in Essex did. The machinists walked out from their jobs making car seat covers as a protest against sexual discrimination while making the demand for equal pay with men. The three-week strike spread to the machinists at the Ford Halewood and Body and Assembly plant in Liverpool and led to the halting of UK Ford car production. The strike was mediated by the Secretary of State for Employment and Productivity, Barbara Castle, and the women returned to work on higher pay. The high profile dispute raised the public's awareness and concern of unequal pay based on gender led to the passing of the 1970 Equal Pay Act (which came in to operation in 1975).

In the following two decades the magazine *Spare Rib*, published by Virago, was to provide women with a vehicle for their increasing demands for equality in all spheres of life. During the 1970s, the women's movement and society's increased awareness of women's position and roles were to play a crucial part in the development of community work. On closer examination we can see that there were three main factors in the development of feminist community work.

First, was the considerable role women played (and continue to play) in the communities or neighbourhoods in which they reside. Despite significant demands for equality in the bringing up of children, women are usually expected to take the main responsibility of child-rearing and are therefore more likely to spend longer periods in their homes and communities than men. Consequently, issues related to their living accommodation, and to the health and welfare of their children and themselves, are closer to their experience than to men's (Mayo 1977; Curno et al. 1982). Second, as seen with the Ford sewing machinists strike, during the late 1960s and early 1970s the issue of the social and economical inequality of women became a public issue. This was due in part to the increased voice of the emerging women's liberation movement; to the developing understanding by many women, and increasingly by men, that women' position was subordinate to that of men's; and to the recognition by the state of women's situation. The outcome was the Equal Pay Act, the Sex Discrimination Act and the establishment of the Equal Opportunities Commission. Third, during the 1960s and early 1970s, community work theory and practice were an activity dominated by white males. The CDPs, which were leading the development of radical community work, were similarly gender-blind. Although the CDPs were working to alleviate poverty, according to a number of writers and activists, they failed to recognize and appreciate the particular concerns of women in poverty (Green and Chapman 1990; Dominelli 2006). However, as the decade progressed, the number of campaigns and organizations initiated and run by women increased. The number of female community workers grew, together with the emergence of the community work literature written by women, and since the 1970s feminist theory has made a significant impact on community work, which we will address further in Chapter 5.

We have noted that a strong push for the establishment of the Urban Programme came from the fear of unrest over the issue of 'race' which was, and still is, a centrally important issue within British society. This was also a factor in the development during the 1960s of the national Community Relations Commission (CRC) and the Race Relations Board. During this period both the CRC and its local equivalents were funding grassroots community work projects and research, which were involved in combating discriminatory treatment of newly settled immigrants and in supporting community groups and organizations.

Finally, much of the growing confidence by minority ethnic groups in the UK to oppose racism came from seeing resistance to racism in the USA. Martin Luther King Jr. and Malcolm X were to lead what became the largest mass movement for racial reform and civil rights during the 1960s and beyond.

State co-option of community work

During the 1970s, the state continued with its drive to improve the inner areas of cities and developed a range of strategies which were aimed at upgrading the physical environment while meeting the needs of people living in certain specified areas. All the above in different ways were to contribute to the development of community work.

The government initiative which was to reshape the physical environment of many urban neighbourhoods was the 1974 Housing Act, which introduced Housing Action Areas and was intended to rehabilitate specified 'deprived areas'. An effect of this legislation was to take the sting out of 'stop the bulldozer' campaigns, with the possibilities of community workers bringing together local authority departments to plan Housing Action Areas on the basis of need, rather than political expediency (Twelvetrees 1983: 31).

With an increase in state-sponsored community work in the 1970s it was perhaps inevitable that many community workers would find themselves in potential and actual conflict with their employers, who were also the providers of the services community groups were criticizing. These dilemmas are discussed in some detail by Cockburn (1977) and the London Edinburgh Weekend Return Group (1980).

The first half of the 1970s was similar to the late 1960s in that a strong theme in community work was its dual role as part of the welfare state while at the same time being critical of the state's inability to reach some of the poorest sections of society. Community work was also critical of the inferior level of public services being offered to the less well off – a matter of poor services for poor people. The guiding premise for many community workers of the period was empowerment, justice and equality. Yet for all the policy statements of the Labour Governments of 1964–70 and 1974–79 committing them to ameliorating poverty and to opening up society to greater equality, little was actually achieved in this direction, which led community workers to experience government as unresponsive and uncaring towards the needs of millions of poor people.

Conclusion

We have seen that community work in the UK has its roots in two conflicting forces that were prevalent in the late nineteenth century. One was in the attempts by Christian organizations, the well-meaning bourgeoisie, and universities to develop the settlement movement, which provided educational and group activities and welfare support to those living in neighbourhoods where poverty was substantial and apparent. This paternalistic approach was also found in work of the British government and its agencies in regions and countries that constituted the British Empire (later titled the British Commonwealth and now the Commonwealth of Nations). The other approach to community work has its roots in local communities and the residents who live there. This direct action was the forerunner of community action and social action, which, as we will see in the following chapter, has come to challenge a number of issues in the UK and elsewhere in more contemporary times. Both traditions of community work (benevolent paternalism and collective community action) have been present in various guises in different periods during its long history.

Community work received a major impetus in the 1960s from a series of international and national events and developments which recharged collective community action to assist in the organization of the poor and disadvantaged in the challenge to economic inequality and social injustice. At the same time, community work became a state-sponsored method of stimulating welfare and education agencies to respond more effectively in what were termed 'pockets of deprivation'. This led to the expansion of community work, with a rapid development during the 1970s of a wide range of activities and styles of working in both the statutory and voluntary sector.

Question
1   What examples are there of the two conflicting roots of community work (benevolent paternalism and community action) that can be identified in the neighbourhood or community that you are familiar with?

4 British community work

The 1970s to the present day

Introduction

In Chapter 3 we traced the early developments in British community work through to the radical influences during the 1960s and increased government funding of the activity in the first half of the 1970s. We commence this chapter by following on from this period and exploring the developments to the present day. Our consideration covers the emergence and impact of the economic and social policies of the New Right, the community-based initiatives of the new Labour government (1997–2010), and then the interventions by the Conservative and Liberal Democratic Coalition government that came to power in 2010 and who made major and sustained attacks on the welfare state and reduced public spending in response to the banking crisis of 2008–09.

The recession of the mid-1970s

A national state of emergency, inflation and public spending cuts

By the mid-1970s, Britain, along with other countries, was beginning to experience an economic recession, due mainly to the aftermath of the Arab–Israeli war of October 1973 which led Arab oil producers to reduce their supplies and increase the price of exported oil. The problem was further compounded by successive governments' deliberate drive to increase Britain's dependence on oil at the expense of home-produced coal. The decision by the National Union of Mineworkers (NUM) to implement a ban on overtime and weekend working from November 1973, in support of a pay claim in excess of the Conservative government's income policy, led to the declaration of a State of Emergency. The NUM called a national miners strike, while the government announced a general election for February 1974. This was not before: public sector cuts of £1.2 million; a rise in the bank minimum lending rate from 4 per cent to 13 per cent; a three-day working week for most industrial workers; the disruption (including the use of mass picketing) of coal deliveries to power stations; and 'a scene of industrial bitterness perhaps unparalleled since the General Strike of 1926' (Sked and Cook 1984: 290). These extraordinary events were to herald the beginnings of a decline in the post-war social-democratic consensus and to create the conditions that were conducive for the rise of the New Right within the Conservative Party which, under the leadership of Margaret Thatcher, was to gain political power five years later.

> The essential launching pad for Thatcherism was the apparent failure of previous governments and previous policies. Fundamental weaknesses in the British economy had not been remedied, while globalization and the power of the money markets intensified the need for strict control of public expenditure.
>
> (Marwick 2000: 268)

The Labour government, 1974–79: community work undergoes a change

The incoming minority Labour government of February 1974 quickly resolved the three-day week and the miners strike and in the following October won a further general election with an increased majority. However, by 1975, the government was presiding over the largest recorded balance-of-payments deficit and rising unemployment and inflation at over 24 per cent. In response, over the next few years further cuts were made in the public sector. However, these measures failed to stem the dramatic slide in the value of sterling and the government was forced to secure a loan from the International Monetary Fund in exchange for increases in taxation and further deep cuts in public expenditure.

The economic crisis of the 1960s was, then, relatively minor compared with the problems facing Britain in the mid-1970s which were to have a marked impact on the development of community work. The most significant feature within community work was the move community workers, together with many other state employees, made from attacking the welfare state to one of defensive struggle. The anti-statism inherent in the philosophy and practice of many community workers was, according to Lees and Mayo (1984: 31), to prove inadequate as a 'basis from which to grapple with the challenge from the anti-statism of monetarists'. Community work became one of the constituents of the welfare state that lost out in the realigned social work and education departments, which were competing for declining real resources. From this period onwards the overriding concern of these departments was to provide statutory or mandatory services. If there was any remaining finance, it was used for non-statutory programmes which could include community work.

Similarly, voluntary organizations that depended upon state support began to experience greater scrutiny of their work and reductions in their funding. Community workers were in some disarray because the emphasis of the state was to finance and support the making of profits in the private sector at the expense of investment in the public sector. This change was to highlight a contradiction within community work which has been well described by Waddington (1983), who argues that social reform had provided the 'baits' which stimulated community work during the 1960s and 1970s. He argued that the removal of these 'baits' was

> a major cause of the falling off of levels of community action and the disorientation of community workers. The plain fact is that many community work activities, as we originally conceived them, have simply lost their point. Our current predicament is that we are no longer collectively quite sure of what we are trying to do or how to do it.
>
> (1983: 43)

Perhaps one of the clearest examples of the dilemmas facing community workers during the 1970s recession was the use of Manpower Services Commission (MSC) schemes to fund the practice. Launched in January 1974 as a means of centralizing responses to growing unemployment, the MSC continually sought ways of reducing the number of people on the unemployment register created by the effects of deindustrialization, while providing low-cost employment and training opportunities for young people and adults. The outcome was a range of schemes, some of which were based in community work projects. The Community Programme, for instance, provided part-time temporary jobs in community settings for the long-term unemployed. The majority of Community Programme workers were male, with more than 65 per cent aged under 25 and most graduates of other unemployment schemes (Finn 1987: 189). This created for many community work practitioners a dilemma they were unable satisfactorily to resolve. One group of community workers argued that the activity should have nothing to do with temporary employment schemes which exploited its participants and which could reduce the opportunities for radical change. The opposing argument accepted the thrust of this position but claimed that local communities needed the resources, the employment and the training offered by the Manpower Services Commission. The key, they argued, was to understand this paradox and secure the best deal possible in the interests of local communities (Jones 1986; Ellison 1988). By the mid-1980s it was estimated that the MSC was the major funder of community work in Britain, but mainstream community workers vigorously pointed out that the meaning of 'community work' as envisaged by the Commission was at variance with that given to it by the activity itself (Hill 1987; Craig 1989).

By the end of the decade the rapid expansion of community work had disappeared. Its swift development through the late 1960s and during the early part of the 1970s was halted by the increasing reductions in public expenditure together with a changing philosophy within society which was emphasizing the need for people to 'stand on their own two feet'. The ascending political creed emphasized self-help and voluntary effort, with projects encouraged to look to the private sector for support and finance.

The New Right and community work

In 1979, under the leadership of Margaret Thatcher, the Conservative Party after the general election made a break with the social-democratic consensus and in its place installed a particular form of potentially authoritarian domination which, according to Hall (1988), threatened to discipline Britain for its own ends. The manifesto on which the Conservatives won the election reflected the thinking and the influence of the New Right, whose advocates included the US economist and Nobel Prize-winner, Professor Milton Friedman, another Nobel Laureate in economics, Professor Friedrich von Hayek, and right-wing 'think tanks', including the Institute of Economic Affairs, the Social Affairs Unit, the Centre for Policy Studies, and the Adam Smith Institute. During the 1979 election campaign the Conservatives exploited the popular discontent with the post-war consensus for welfare, health, education and housing, and promised to reverse the relative decline in the British economy and in the values which they argued were affecting Britain's ability to address its future destiny. To quote Thatcher reflecting on this time:

> I believe that five years ago the British people made me Prime Minister primarily because they sensed that socialism had been leading them a life of debilitating dependency on the state, when what they really wanted was the independence and freedom of self-reliance and responsibility.
>
> (*Financial Times*, 24 July 1986)

In fact, Thatcher launched the UK's neo-liberal economic policies and practices that have since come to dominate the national and international scene and which we first discussed in Chapter 1.

The key principles enshrined in what became known as Thatcherism were: the primacy of wealth creation; the regulation of distribution through market principles, accompanied by the notion of individual rather than public choice; the redistribution of income and wealth based upon the 'trickle-down' theory; an attack on, and a restructuring of, the state's welfare responsibilities; the comprehensive deregulation of large areas of public and private activity;

an assault on the influence of the trade union movement; and the notion of absolute poverty as opposed to relative poverty.

Although the Thatcher government was hostile to the welfare state and collectivism, the first years of its period in office were spent changing the priorities and the emphases rather than mounting an overt attack on the post-war creation. For instance, the government encouraged private education and health care and introduced the sale of council houses to tenants. However, according to Walker (1987: 1), what was beginning on a broader scale was the government's 'indifference and, in some instances, outright antagonism towards poor families and the social services on which they depend'.

This indifference and antagonism were believed to be a feature of the Thatcher government's attitude towards the poor and the welfare state, and was evidenced by the increasing poverty and unemployment; by an increasing divide between the rich and the poor and between those living in the 'North' and the 'South' in the UK; by a growth in the impoverishment of women and ethnic minorities; and by encouraging growth in the stigmatization and marginalization of claimants. It was argued that the creation of this more sharply divided society was an essential component of the social and economic policies pursued by the government in its desire to institute a 'sound economy based on free enterprise and individual family responsibility' (Walker 1987: 1).

While the rise of the New Right was accompanied by an economic recession which was borne disproportionately by the poor, advocates of the New Right found that their theory did not produce the outcomes they had expected and instead resulted in a continuation of Britain's economic decline. One commentator described this in the following way:

> Public expenditure and taxation have been restructured but not reduced. A very large income transfer towards the upper income groups has been engineered with a corresponding significant increase in poverty. There has been an enormous shake-out of labour but few signs of the permanent increase in productivity needed to improve competitiveness.
>
> (Gamble 1987: 199)

So the Conservative government did not perform the promised economic miracle. In fact the gross national product of Britain grew less during the Thatcher period than in the 1950s, 1960s and 1970s, and Britain became the first industrial nation to import more manufactured goods than it exported (Coutts and Godley 1989; Johnson 1991). However, New Right thinking had a significant impact upon the welfare state during the 1980s and in turn had implications for the development of community work.

The growth of 'community work' under Thatcherism

Despite the influence of New Right thinking in the Thatcher government, community work enjoyed an expansion during the 1980s. A survey undertaken in 1983 of community workers in the United Kingdom indicated that 5,000 practitioners were employed at the time, compared with little more than 1,000 in the early 1970s (Francis et al. 1984). One commentator believes this increase was due to: many agencies re-designating jobs and adding the term 'community' to their titles; the state's policy of community care and the resultant 'layer of workers, albeit low-paid, to implement its strategy of shifting the burden of welfare work from public collective to private individual shoulders' (Craig 1989: 12); and to the growth in the number of workers required to operate a battery of Manpower Services Commission employment schemes.

The 1980s were distinguished by the government's push to encourage the development of strategies in the community for the care of older people and people with disabilities while cutting expenditure on health and social services (Wagner 1988; DHSS 1989). A central aspect of the New Right philosophy was the need for welfare services to demonstrate increased efficiency and effectiveness before being allocated further public funds. Meanwhile the state encouraged the voluntary and private sectors to fill the vacuum (Iliffe 1985). It was in this changed context that community work found itself being employed.

Community social work

During the 1980s a philosophy and practice of community social work developed within social work which drew on pluralist community work ideas of working in small areas called 'patches', and from the skills acquired through working with informal networks (Barclay 1982; Hadley et al. 1987). Established in a number of local authorities, social work teams employed the community social work approach while setting up 'self-help' groups and organizations, community care schemes, and by encouraging a range of voluntary organizations, including the settlements, to provide a social work service at a reduced cost per client. Community work in this context became used by local authorities to discharge its responsibilities for caring for its citizens within a budget limited by central government. In the process of encouraging community work, the state ensured that the activity's boundaries were closely drawn in an attempt to avoid the experiences it had encountered during the 1970s when the CDPs criticized the state for its role in supporting the excesses of capitalism.

Inner-city riots

Meanwhile, during the 1980s, community work, in its more traditional role, was frequently used by the state as a means of intervening at the neighbourhood level to dampen social and political unrest. The violent disorder in a number of British urban areas during 1980, 1981, 1985 and 1986 was thought by a number of writers, including Benyon and Solomos (1987), to have its roots in unemployment, deprivation, racism, political exclusion and police malpractices. The feeling of many young people living in disadvantaged circumstances was that government programmes were failing to meet their needs and they therefore felt they had little stake in society or its institutions.

At the time of the disorders the government appointed a Cabinet committee to examine inner-city policy and the Urban Programme, so giving the overall appearance that it was dealing with the issues raised by them. The government also appointed a 'Minister for Merseyside', Michael Heseltine, the Environment Secretary, who was given the task of regenerating one of the areas, Toxteth in Liverpool, that had experienced rioting. Little else was undertaken by the state other than a public inquiry into the riots in Brixton, south London, which produced the Scarman Report (HMSO 1981). This report made a number of recommendations in relation to the role and training of the police, who in response claimed they were developing more effective means of handling future disorders. Throughout this period the Urban Programme and the Inner City Partnership schemes were used to fund local community projects in areas that experienced unrest. Community work was again employed as a palliative when the substantial resources needed to overcome the major injustices were not forthcoming.

The role of the Manpower Services Commission

The MSC continued to be a major funder of community work during the decade, with Smith (1989) providing evidence that it was spending over £8 million on community projects in Sheffield, while the local authority spent only £1.5 million on community work. As the main funder of welfare workers in the city, the Commission issued an instruction to workers to refrain from engaging in welfare rights campaign work. This control of community work to ensure projects' 'political neutrality' impacted on a number of community workers dependent on state funding. Similarly, reductions in local and central government budgets led to a decline in many local community resource centres which were often pivotal in community struggles over housing, health and women's issues (*Community Action*, 83, Spring 1990).

Community work in the 1990s: the changing world

In the Spring of 1990, the final issue of *Community Action* was published. This national magazine, a brightly burning beacon in the community work field for almost 20 years, finally succumbed to the exhaustion of its voluntary workers and a decline in resources for radical community work. The magazine was absorbed into *Public Service Action*, published by Services to Community Action and Tenants. The closure of this independent, non-profit-making magazine was a significant and symbolic event in the community work field and reflected the changing world that community work was now moving into.

Responsibility for the various programmes for the unemployed were devolved by the government in the early 1990s from its own agency to 82 regional Training and Enterprise Councils in England and Wales and 22 Local Enterprise Councils in Scotland. These councils, which were managed by directors of large private firms, with only a minor involvement by education-alists, unions and local authorities, were part of a drive to encourage employers to take further financial and practical responsibility for training future workers. The trend of moving state services into the private sector has continued to the present day. The Community Programme, which was an important source of funding for different forms of community work, was disbanded. In its place the government introduced a 'Community Action Programme', intended to provide 60,000 part-time 'community work places' for those people unemployed for more than a year (Weston 1993).

The impact of the Poll Tax

The Community Charge (widely known as the poll tax), which was introduced in Scotland in April 1989, and in England and Wales a year later, proved to be one of the most unpopular taxes of modern times. The flat-rate local tax led to wealthy and poor people alike receiving similar tax demands. In response, one of the largest mass movements in British history, which at its peak involved over 17 million people, formed to demonstrate and protest against what was considered to be a major injustice. The effects of the tax were far-reaching, with many people

> [having] to pay bills which were two or three times higher than before. This was because the costs of administration were twice as high and because dramatic reductions in the tax bills of the wealthy were paid for by ordinary people.
>
> (Burns 1992: 10)

Local authorities came under increasing financial pressure as large numbers of people withheld all or part of their tax, and those councils that budgeted for more expenditure than central government permitted faced rate-capping. In an attempt to keep within budgets, local authorities reduced a number of their services, including resources for community work (Taylor 1992: 15).

The creation of business-led local authorities

The changes local authorities underwent in the 1980s continued in the 1990s as local government was being transformed to fit into a new business-led provider of welfare (Butcher et al. 1990; Cochrane 1993). The developments in care in the community following the 1990 National Health Service and Community Care Act reflected this trend and, according to one observer, were to offer us 'a striking Thatcherite synthesis of the free market' (Langan 1990: 59). The role undertaken by local authorities in the 1990s from April 1993, when community care legislation came into force, was that of service enabler. With new funding arrangements, local authorities contracted in various welfare functions and services, with community organizations and groups, along with private care agencies, competing to provide them. This ideological and practical shift was thought by some to assist in redressing the balance between professionals and the public, with Taylor (1992: 20) arguing that community development had 'an important role in making this work'. The concern was that community work was being used to offer low-cost strategies to tackle problems that demanded substantial resources.

Sins of the fathers

During the 1990s, industry and commerce in the United Kingdom continued to suffer from problems of under-investment and a large trade imbalance with the rest of the world. According to many economists, the UK was paying the price of poor economic management during the 1980s. To quote the Economics Editor of the *Guardian*:

> The sins of the fathers have truly been visited upon the sons. The 1980's, the decade of the economic miracle, was in reality 10 years of wild economic mismanagement and monstrous self-delusion. Britain over-consumed and under-produced to an astonishing degree and has been left with its finances – private, public and external – in such disarray that it may take the whole of the 1990's to recover. And even that is not certain.
>
> (Hutton 1993)

With official unemployment rates at around 2.5 million, but 'real' unemployment 1 million higher (Unemployment Unit and Youth Aid 1993), new social and economic divisions, a growing elderly and dependent population, and 'opting out' and contracting of local authority services, there appeared to be fresh contemporary challenges for the activity known as community work.

1997–2010 New Labour and community participation

As we noted in Chapter 1, New Labour, under the leadership of Tony Blair, were elected to government in May 1997 with a 'landslide' 179-seat majority. Many hoped that the incoming government would steer a radical path away from the economic policies of the Conservative administration. However, in a short time it became clear that New Labour planned to keep faith with the neo-liberal ideology of the Margaret Thatcher and John Major Conservative governments. Nevertheless the Labour government attempted through the welfare benefit system to raise the standard of living for poorer families with young children, and those of pensionable age. They introduced a legally enforceable minimum wage, cut the level of VAT on heating bills, reduced school class sizes for primary aged children, took young people off welfare benefits by introducing a windfall tax on privatized utilities to pay for their training, and introduced targets for NHS waiting times by shifting resources away from administration to frontline medical services.

Capacity building and the New Deal for Communities

To its credit, the Labour government emphasized and articulated the values of community, inclusion and opportunity whilst investing heavily in health services, education and launched a number of area-based regeneration projects such as Sure Start for children, and the New Deal for Communities that attempted to address problems facing identified disadvantaged neighbourhoods. Community participation was a key aspect of both projects.

Perhaps most importantly for community work at this time was a change in the rhetoric used in the field. One of the key moves was into capacity building which was often tied to economic development, something that is prevalent in community work in the USA. Capacity building has been described by Skinner (1997: 1–2) as development work that

> strengthens the ability of community organizations and groups to build their structures, systems, people and skills so that they are better able to define and achieve their objectives and engage in consultation and planning, manage community projects and take part in partnerships and community enterprises.

The regeneration programme, New Deal for Communities (NDC), launched by New Labour in 1998 was a further attempt by a British government to tackle problems in some of England's most disadvantaged neighbourhoods and encourage capacity building. The NDCs which encompassed some 39 neighbourhoods (10 of which were in London) were an attempt to respond to the concerns of residents of local communities (each with around 9,900 population) regarding crime, a sense of community, housing and the physical environment, health, education and lack of jobs. Each local NDC had approximately £50 million to spend over a ten-year period in an attempt to both transform the neighbourhoods and to 'close the gaps' between the 39 areas and the rest of the country. The NDCs were an even more concerted (and better funded) attempt than the NCDP of the late 1960s and 1970s to deliver a neighbourhood intervention that placed the notion of community at its core. The Final Assessment of the NDC makes a number of useful observations on the community dimension of the Programme, including the statement that 'communities can play an especially strong role in defining needs and validating the additionality of new proposals emerging from mainstream delivery agencies' (Batty et al. 2010: 4).

The effects of social exclusion were considered to be a significant weakness of the neo-liberal economic policies that New Labour was pursuing and the government made attempts to address this with a plethora of social policies and commitments by the Social Exclusion Unit aimed at aiding community cohesion and preventing violent extremism in deprived neighbourhoods. Lister (2001) provides a valuable analysis of these initiatives and suggests that though they reflected some acknowledgement of the challenges facing the poor in these areas by increasing resources, New Labour failed to satisfactorily address the far reaching and damaging economic and social problems confronting such neighbourhoods. So while community work was a valuable tool in the armoury of New Labour's attack on deprivation, the continuous policy activity over the period from 1997 to 2010 made only the smallest of inroads in producing positive results. Supporting the judgements of Lister (2001), Syrett and North (2010: 477) argue that successive New Labour governments

> struggled both to confront the economic basis of the problems of deprived neighbourhoods and to put in place the necessary governance arrangements to tackle the problem. The result was a plethora of initiatives and an ever-changing governance landscape which, although it produced some significant localized impacts, did not provide the basis for any widespread reversal in the economic fortunes of deprived neighbourhoods.

Rural community work

Attention is usually given to urban community work which appears to consume the majority of resources and support from funders. However, in 2004, the Carnegie UK Trust launched its *Commission of Inquiry into the Future of Community Development in Rural Areas*. This led to the Trust developing and running between 2008 and 2012 the Fiery Spirits Rural Development Community of Practice in partnership with the Highlands and

Islands Enterprise. This network brought together activists and professionals who exchanged information on how they had built vibrant, resilient rural communities. In 2013, the Trust announced the Plunkett Foundation would become the new host of Fieryspirits.com, taking on the commitment and support of this area of work.

The global economic crisis 2008–09

In 2007, Tony Blair stood down from his position as Prime Minister, as an MP and formally left the House of Commons. The in-coming Prime Minister, Gordon Brown, who as the Chancellor of the Exchequer had acknowledged and commended the neo-liberal economic policies and had declared that regulation in the City of London would require only 'a light touch', was within a year in office faced with leading the UK's response to what turned out to be a global economic crisis.

To place this crisis in context, we need to recognize that during the late 1970s and the 1980s unemployment and free-market reforms reduced the power of the UK's industrial labour force as investment was moved from manufacturing industries and into the finance sector. Between 1997 and 2007 some 80 per cent of the investment in the UK was 'in financial products and mortgages' (Jordan and Drakeford 2012: 25). To quote the Economics Editor of the *Guardian*:

> Financial capitalism delivered higher profits, but only by suppressing wages. But since market economies can only function if there is sufficient demand for goods and services, a way had to be found to boost consumption. That was achieved through higher levels of personal debt, cheerfully provided by the newly liberalized financial services sector. Growth rates were kept artificially high, and the tax revenues thereby generated allowed governments to spend more than they could actually afford. To complete the picture, the debt was shifted across national borders by globalization, so China would lend America the money to buy the cheap industrial products being made in the factories of east Asia, and Germany would do the same for the less competitive members of the eurozone.
>
> (Elliott 2012)

While many economists and commentators will point to the overall weakness of the UK economy prior to 2008, in that year it became apparent that the collapse of the US sub-prime mortgage market, the U-turn in the housing boom in many industrialized countries, and the exposure of the weaknesses in the global financial systems were leading to a lack of confidence in the banking system. On the back of an economic boom, UK high street banks had engaged in a form of investment banking and were trading in often high risk schemes. As it became clear that the UK-based banks had debts that were greater than their assets and were financially insolvent, they turned to the government for substantial financial support. If the government had not 'bailed' them out, many businesses in the UK would have been driven to the wall and millions of individuals would not have been able to access their personal money. The outcome was that the government covered the banks' enormous losses and took a part in their ownership.

2010 onwards: austerity and the 'Big Society'

It was plain to most people living in the UK that soon after the May 2010 General Election the incoming Conservative-led Coalition government had a completely different vision of how to organize public services and society than the outgoing Labour administration.

The Coalition government was created with an agreement between the Conservative Party and the Liberal Democratic Party to share power. While the Conservatives received the largest number of votes in the general election, and secured the largest number of seats in Parliament, they were 20 seats short of a majority and could not rule without support from the LibDems who had won 57 seats.

Faced with a major deficit in the public finances due to the shoring-up the previous government had to make to the banks, the incoming Conservative-led Coalition government made significant cuts in the country's health, education, housing and social care services in order to reduce the debt and arguably in doing so undid much of the social progress made by the previous Labour government. For example, the Coalition substantially raised university student tuition fees, launched an attack on welfare claimants, and reduced the finance given to local authorities, which led to a significant reduction in their services to local communities.

The 'Big Society': a flagship policy idea and its critics

In July 2010, alongside the launch of the Coalition's economic austerity programme, the Prime Minister David Cameron initiated one of his flagship policy ideas for England. Termed the 'Big Society', it was based on the work of Blond (2010), the political commentator and author of *Red Tory* (2010), whose book argues that people should take more responsibility for their own welfare and be encouraged to volunteer in their local communities. The thrust of Cameron's policy idea was to repair what he claimed was Britain's 'broken society'. Arguing that the top-down targets and solutions approach of New Labour was impeding the positive forces that made society work, Cameron saw the voluntary sector and in particular co-operatives, mutual, charities and social enterprises taking a more active role in providing services so as to help people come together in order to participate more fully in their neighbourhoods. This role was intended to supplement the work of local and national government, which he wanted to demonstrate greater openness and transparency. A key aim of the 'Big Society' has been to encourage volunteerism through the training of community organizers and the funding of community groups by the Community First Programme which is delivered through the Community Development Foundation. The aim of this Programme is to support communities to enable them to build more self-confidence and capability so that they can make changes in their areas.

Despite the positive spin the Coalition government has given the 'Big Society', there have been a number of high profile criticisms of its work. For example, Dr Rowan Williams, who was Archbishop of Canterbury at the time (June 2011), questioned the notion of the 'Big Society' in a leader article in the *New Statesman* (Williams 2011), while Dame Elisabeth Hoodless, who was retiring as Director of the Community Service Volunteers, claimed that there was no strategic plan to the 'Big Society' and what she termed 'massive' cuts in council budgets would make it harder for people to get involved in their communities (www.bbc.co.uk/news/uk-politics-12378974. accessed 21 August 2013).

The government's enthusiasm for the 'Big Society' has to be placed against the substantial cuts they have made to the funding of the voluntary and community sector which in turn has decreased the services they can deliver (Skills-Third Sector 2013). So while the voluntary and community sector can make a considerable contribution to neighbourhood life, as well as making contact with 'hard-to-reach' groups, their finances are shrinking at the very time they are expected by central government to fill the gap left by central government funding cuts. There is therefore a disparity between what community organizations can provide and the declining funding available to undertake this task. For example, a 2011 member survey by Community Matters, which is the national umbrella body for community associations and similar multi-purpose community organizations in the UK, showed that its members were struggling to meet the increasing demand for their services. The survey revealed that member income had dropped by 18 per cent from 2010, and many organizations were living on their reserves which also dropped by 29 per cent in the same period. The main areas that had suffered disproportionately from cuts in public expenditure were in youth provision and arts and cultural activity (Community Matters 2011).

Community Action

Since 2010, there has been a marked increase in community and social action in the UK. Much of this increase has been in an angry response to the financial reductions in the public sector mentioned above, to concerns about increasing environmental degradation, and to disillusion with the impact of the political parties and the mendacity of politicians. For example, Nick Clegg, the LibDem leader promised in the 2010 General Election campaign he would not support the raising of university student tuition fees but did just that when becoming Deputy Prime Minister. David Cameron said in the same campaign that if in power he would not raise Value Added Tax (VAT) but did raise the tax level when in government. Cameron also promised not to reduce frontline services but then oversaw the removal of 6,000 nurses, 10,000 police officers and 10,000 teachers (Toynbee 2013). In response to these reversals in promises, Toynbee questions in the same article whether anyone will believe any political party at the next UK general election.

A good deal of the more recent self-organized community action has been focused in local areas and has involved campaigns to challenge established public and private sector bodies.

For example, there have been numerous campaigns to prevent the closure of libraries www.campaignengineroom.org.uk/save-our-libraries (accessed 7 January 2014). It is estimated local authority cut-backs due to the government's austerity measures could lead to the closure of 400 libraries, with the loss of some 6,000 librarian posts. Libraries are thought by many to be a source of social and community life and their closure impacts on people's sense of community. Libraries too are important for their internet facilities, which are an important resource for those who do not have internet access at home.

Campaigns by people living in small rural communities and attempting to maintain their sense of community are also prevalent in the present times. For example, villagers in Brechfa in Carmarthenshire, Wales (pop. 300) who run a community shop, tried unsuccessfully to take ownership of their empty local pub, and who saw their chapel closed in 2011, have been campaigning to keep the primary school from closing. The villagers' plan is to develop the school as an educational facility, community centre and to develop business units on the premises. As one of the campaigners said:

> To be a sustainable village; you need a school, a pub, a post office and a shop and gradually we've lost all those things. Salvaging the shop has helped community life but we still need somewhere for people to meet and greet each other.
> (www.walesonline.co.uk/news/wales-news/welsh-villagers-plead-help-save-2496650, accessed 8 January 2014)

The other area of concern where we have witnessed community action has been by members of local communities who have been challenging the growth of hydraulic fracturing or fracking, which involves the process of drilling and injecting fluid into the ground at high pressure in order to fracture shale rocks which then release natural gas. Advocates of fracking have pointed to the process producing substantial energy sources at low cost. Local communities have, however, argued the development of fracking has produced adverse environmental effects, including the pollution of underground water, the depletion of fresh water, air and noise pollution and the health impact of the gases released and the hydraulic chemicals used in the process. While fracking has a long history in the USA, the activity has been banned and restricted by the French and German governments, nevertheless international companies have been using the technique in the North Sea since the early 1980s and are presently carrying out testing on the UK mainland. Opposition to fracking has come from a national group called 'Frack Off', however, local community groups in the UK have engaged in protests in their areas to raise the issue which has received national publicity.

Social networks and social movements

While in recent years there have been a considerable number of localized campaigns, protests and examples of community action throughout the UK, it is important to mention that new forms of social movements have appeared both in Britain and throughout a good deal of the world.

It is argued by scholars and commentators such as Castells (2012) and Mason (2012) that the Arab uprisings (or the Arab Spring) from December 2010 onwards which have included protests, strikes, riots and civil wars were due to dissatisfaction with local and national governments, political corruption, dictatorships and absolute monarchy, human rights violations, unemployment and the income disparity between the small group of the extremely wealthy, the majority of people on average incomes, and those in extreme poverty. However, what has made these forms of activism different from those in previous generations is the use of personal communication technology which in an instant has connected individuals with others, so forming oppositional groups and movements. Both Castells and Mason argue that digital networks offer the opportunities for communities everywhere to enjoy largely unfettered discussion and co-ordination in their campaigns. This is in response to the mass media which is mainly controlled by governments and mass media corporations.

Similarly, participants in the Occupy Movement, the international protest group established to highlight social and economic inequality, have benefited from the use of Facebook, Twitter and Meetup to co-ordinate events throughout the world. These new forms of social media are likely to be further used by local groups as they organize protests and campaigns.

Conclusion

We have seen that the state became a major funder of community work in the 1960s and 1970s. However, with the establishment of New Right philosophy and policies in the late 1970s and early 1980s, community work found its scope, focus and direction determined by a rigid doctrine which clashed with the traditionally liberal, and in many cases socialist and radical, views and ideals of its practitioners. In the 1990s, community work was dealing with the decline of the Urban Programme, changes in the employment training schemes, and the introduction of schemes brought in by the Labour government to tackle social exclusion. All these had an impact on community work activity.

Contemporary community work is therefore at a significant stage in its evolution which reflects the continuing tension between consensus and in some examples regressive practice, and collective community action, much of which is linked to wider concerns with social and economic justice. What we have emerging is a tussle between two approaches to community issues. One is to engage in strategies which have at their centre what can be termed vertical politics with the emphasis on voting, and working with local and central government to achieve change. The other approach favours direct community action and can be termed horizontal politics. However, for many, a combination of both approaches is needed.

In the last two chapters we have noted the increasing influence of the state in the development of community work. In the present period the state remains influential but as we have seen there is increasing evidence that community work is emphasizing its more radical roots which we will examine in more detail in the following chapters.

Questions

It has been argued that contemporary state-funded community work has been shaped to meet the needs of communities to deal with the impact of neo-liberal economic and social policies.

1   What are the tensions facing those employed in this area of work? How might they be resolved?
2   Community action is presently using the development of social media sites and digital technology. What are the benefits of these new forms of communication for community action? What are the pitfalls?

---

5   Community work theories

Introduction

In the previous two chapters we have reflected on how British community work has evolved over the last century or more. This examination enabled us to locate the activity alongside the changing social, economic and political landscape both in the UK and internationally. This chapter further helps us to understand and analyse community work more effectively by exploring the nature of the different theories or categories of theoretical knowledge that inform the activity. After a short discussion on the meaning of theory, we will consider the diverse key perspectives and their relation to community work. We conclude the chapter with an evaluation of these theoretical debates.

What is theory and why is it important?

The term *theory* is an integral feature of social science investigation and is employed to explain social phenomena. However, the term itself is rarely examined. It is therefore valuable to briefly consider what the term means before exploring the various theories that inform community work. In this chapter we will also use the term *theoretical knowledge* which is essentially the same as the concept of *theory*.

On a basic level, humans not only 'do things' but also think about what they are doing. They attempt to make sense of their encounters with the world, to look for patterns and regularities in order to predict the outcome of their actions. Generally we seek to reduce the uncertainty in the material and social world by creating ideas and theories which are then tested and become established, the overall purpose being to create a greater understanding of the world which we inhabit and to make our encounters and interactions less threatening.

Although a theory is a system of ideas or statements that explains a group of facts or phenomena, theories themselves are neither totally objective nor ahistorical. For instance, the biological theories of 'race' which were created in the nineteenth century claimed that it was possible to classify the different human 'races' by their physical characteristics, in particular, skin colour. From this classification biologists argued that some 'races' were superior to others, and later in the century, under the influence of Darwin's theory of evolution, it was believed this difference was the consequence of the process of natural selection. These theories are now refuted, and are seen as attempts to support the view that white people are superior to black people. However, when the theories were in existence, they were given powerful legitimation by white society which benefited from the results of these theories in practice. Further, it is possible to argue that nearly all the disciplines that inform our understanding of social relations and human behaviour were originally based on Western assumptions of the world, and were deployed to sustain dominant cultural understandings and beliefs.

Theories or theoretical knowledge, therefore, have to be treated with caution and understood as a feature of the society and the period in which they are located. Despite these reservations, having an understanding of the different theoretical strands that inform community work is essential if we are to have a basis for action. As we noted in Chapter 1, community work draws on a number of diverse disciplines, including economics, sociology, social policy, social and economic history, and political science. Community work has developed and adapted these perspectives in order to understand the problems facing communities and to consider effective ways of intervening to address these.

Over the years there have been a number of reviews of the development of theory in British community work (see, for example, Bryers 1979; Hanmer and Rose 1980; Tasker 1980; Thomas 1983; Craig et al. 2011; Gilchrist and Taylor 2011). These studies conclude that there is no distinct community work theory, rather a clutch of theories which can broadly be divided into categories related to macro-theories of society. The categories used in this work are: pluralist theories; radical and socialist theories; feminist theories; the ethnic minority and anti-racist critique; and theories relating to environmentalism and the green movement.

With this in mind, and taking account of Howe's comment below, we can now examine the theories that have made a contribution to community work.

> Theories are not absolute notions of the way things really are, but, so long as they account for what appears to be happening in a particular way that satisfies the observer, they are retained. Theories provide 'workable definitions' of the world about us. They make it intelligible. In a very real way, theory-building is reality building . . . Our theories define what we see.
>
> (Howe 1987: 10)

Pluralist theories

As we observed earlier, pluralist theories have dominated the debate around modern community work since the early 1960s. Furthermore, as we noted in the previous two chapters on the development of community work, pluralism has been an integral aspect of the social-democratic politics which was in the ascendancy during the post-war period.

Pluralist theories, which have been strongly influenced by Weber (1930; 1978), argue that power in modern Western liberal democracies is not located in any single group or type of group. Instead, in a democracy, all public policies are the outcome of compromises between different competing groups. Pluralist theories claim that no group that wishes to affect outcomes lacks the necessary resources, and each may therefore be effective on some issues. It is argued that these competing interest groups or factions are seen as vital to democracy and stability because they divide power and prevent any one group or class exerting an exclusive influence. This continual bargaining between the numerous interest groups in society means they all have some impact on policy. According to pluralist theories, the state has a role in balancing these different competing interests and ensuring that political decision-making takes account of the range of views expressed by the electorate.

In relation to community work, pluralist theories suggest a role that is active in supporting and encouraging participation in the political and administrative processes as a means of increasing the accessibility and accountability of services. Historically, pluralist theories have been linked with mainstream social administration, with their concern for intervention in the shape of piecemeal reforms and the amelioration of social problems. The role of community work in this paradigm is to help various groups to overcome the problems they face in their neighbourhoods or communities, often through mutual support, sharing activities, and by attempting to secure better services for their members.

One of the early attempts to develop a community work practice theory in Britain was by Batten (1967), whose work was influenced by pluralist theories. A former community development worker in ex-colonies, Batten constructed an educational approach that aimed at personal growth. This practice theory argued that by working towards people's self-direction and responsibility, it was possible for them to change their attitudes and responses which in turn would lead to an improvement in their material conditions. This approach, which informed much of the early community work training, was later to attract criticism from more radical approaches.

As we noted in previous chapters, the practice theories of community work based on a pluralist analysis have been developed over the years by a number of writers, including Biddle and Biddle (1965), Goetschius (1975), Henderson and Thomas (2013), Leaper (1971), Thomas (1983) and Twelvetrees (2008). Thomas, for instance, argues that community work is a pluralist occupation and that the political differences that exist within community worker groups are a strength, but that 'we need to create the organisational and conceptual basis around which differences might cohere within a reasonably evident occupational identity' (Thomas 1983: 16). Later he describes community work as a 'public service occupation, with a discernible set of skills and knowledge' (Thomas 1983: 231).

Although primarily concerned with theories of community work practice as opposed to 'grand theories' of society, the pluralist approach nevertheless acknowledges the structural nature of deprivation and recognizes the political dimension to community work. The focus, however, is on micro-change, since advocates of this approach believe that community work is concerned with social consensus and marginal improvements, and hence they emphasize the value of its educational and experimental aspects. In this context, education is seen as a means of 'enhancing political responsibility', the equipping of groups and individuals for effective participation, and, to quote one of its main exponents, 'the promotion and maintenance of communal coherence – the repair of social networks, the awakening of consciousness and responsibility for others and the creation of roles and functions that provide individual significance and a social service' (Thomas 1983: 97). Pluralist theories lay considerable stress upon the importance of skills, and although recognizing the centrality of values, good practice is defined in terms of technical competence rather than conformance to any particular set of values: 'We suggest that there are identifiable skills and techniques which can be used in a multiplicity of situations regardless of the theoretical or ideological stance of workers or neighbourhood groups' (Henderson and Thomas 2013: 31).

An example of pluralist theory and its application to community work

Skills in Neighbourhood Work, 4th edition (Henderson and Thomas 2013) is not only a 'how-to-do-it' text but also a clear exposition of the pluralist approach to community work. It emphasizes the need to focus on the neighbourhood because this is where people are increasingly spending their time due to changes in work patterns, including unemployment; due to demographic changes, including an increasingly older population; and due to policy initiatives, for instance, the move from institutional care to community care. The authors argue that there exists a poverty of neighbourhood theory due to the emphasis in community work on the 'vertical relationships between community groups and resource holders' rather than 'an interest in community interaction' (Henderson and Thomas 2013: 19). As we will see later, this is clearly a reference to the radical and socialist approaches to community work. The text supports the view that neighbourhoods need professional workers skilled in working with people to achieve what the authors describe as 'community capability'. Henderson and Thomas write with a view to encouraging other professionals, including social workers, youth workers and education workers, as well as community development workers, to adopt neighbourhood-based work. The aim of the text therefore is to assist community workers, and in particular neighbourhood workers, to develop a repertoire of skills and knowledge to accomplish a wide range of tasks.

Radical and socialist theories

As we noted earlier, the late 1960s and early 1970s witnessed the emergence of community work theories based upon radical and socialist thinking. Radical theories of society have traditionally advocated far-reaching and fundamental changes in the political, social and economic system. A radical has been described as someone 'who proposes to attack some political or social problem by going deep into the socio-economic fabric to get at the fundamental or root cause and alter this basic social weakness' (Robertson 1985: 80). Radical theories include anarchism, which is based on the proposition that society can operate without a government, and that governments are only legitimate if they are truly consented to by the individuals they govern. Anarchism advocates the establishment and the operation of voluntary associations based on co-operative principles and mutual aid. Radical theories, including anarchism, have often been associated with the Far Left in the political spectrum, and are used as such in the context here. However, it should be noted that it is possible to talk in political terms of the radical centre and the radical right, and to recognize that anarchists have been associated with the Far Right. Finally, Fromm (1969) believes radicalism need not relate to a set of ideas but to an attitude or approach where everything is questioned or doubted.

Socialism, on the other hand, has come to mean a variety of different things. At its most basic it is a political-economic system where the state controls, to a greater or less degree, the means of production in order to produce what is necessary for and needed by society without regard to the desire to obtain a profit. The central features of socialism include the creation of a just and egalitarian society, the removal of poverty, and the establishment of a particular moral system. Internationally, socialism as a political ideal is underpinned by a Marxist critique of capitalism. In the United Kingdom, socialism has come to mean an ideology based on both Fabianism and Marxism. Fabianism, which dates from 1884 and which has always been closely related to the British Labour Party, has traditionally advocated a peaceful political progress to socialism, through electoral politics. According to Alcock et al. (2008: 33), the Fabian Society of the nineteenth and twentieth centuries believed

> Socialism in Britain was entirely compatible with the institutions of the state and could, and should, be realized through a parliamentary route. The state itself, they held, could be harnessed to promote the

collective good and act as a neutral umpire between the demands of different interests.

The radical and socialist theories emerged in community work in the late 1960s. These theories were used by community workers to understand inequality within society, and the disadvantage experienced by a range of individuals and groups. As Britain's manufacturing base declined, particularly in older industrial and inner-city areas, and while rapid industrial change occurred elsewhere, working-class communities began to experience great difficulties. This led community workers to advocate and develop community action which supported groups and communities in conflict with authority. In a seminal paper on the origins of the radical trend within community work, Baldock (1977) argues that radicals and socialists were able to put into practice their developing theories because of: the expansion of community work during the 1960s and 1970s; the ideological influences and the political and social upheaval in the late 1960s, which encouraged critical rethinking of consensus and conservative views of society (both these points were discussed in Chapters 3 and 4); and the receptivity of 'target areas' for more radical community work practice, especially in projects related to slum clearance. Community work practice that has been informed by these theories has traditionally been undertaken by community activists who have employed a class analysis and the rhetoric and pursuance of class struggle at both a local and regional level. These theories have encouraged community work activity outside state funding, although one of the most notable examples of community workers using radical and socialist theories were those employed in the state-funded Community Development Projects.

Later the work of Gough (1979) and the London Edinburgh Weekend Return Group (1980) applied a Marxist political economy approach to an analysis of the welfare state. This analysis highlighted the contradictory nature of the welfare state and its contradictory impact upon capitalism. The authors argue that the welfare state contains policies that can be defended and extended, while recognizing, exposing and attacking its negative aspects. In this way, they argue, 'welfare capitalism' can be transformed into 'welfare socialism'. These theories were to lead radical and socialist community workers to recognize the value of engaging in the activity as state-funded employees and trying to find the oppositional space to undertake work that successfully sustains a struggle against the state. This has been described as a 'progressive form of practice' (Bolger et al. 1981: 144).

Since the 1990s, there has been widespread recognition that socialism as a system has 'failed' in the former Soviet Union and in eastern European countries. These countries had a one-party communist political system which controlled both the economic sphere and the political structures. However, from 1989 onwards, dramatic events in these regions led to the established regimes being replaced by quasi-forms of democracy which, while still highly regulated, have provided space for independent political parties and movements. For example, in Russia during 2012, we saw the emergence of the feminist conceptual punk bank Pussy Power, the members of which received prison sentences in August of that year for what was considered to be a provocative one-minute performance in front of a small audience in Moscow's Cathedral of Christ the Saviour. Members of the band have claimed they formed in anger against President Putin's elitist and corrupt rule. In turn, Pussy Power have gathered support internationally with people applauding their courage and commitment in the face of oppressive state power.

Finally, it is argued that Marx's predictions of worker revolutions in the economically advanced, industrialized societies of the West have not happened, which has posed a dilemma for advocates of the socialist ideal. Whether socialism will again attract the popular appeal it did in the past is uncertain, although, as Scase (1992) has argued, Marxist theory continues to be relevant in contemporary society, providing us with a valuable critique of industrial capitalism, class relations, inequality and the causes of poverty. Marxist theory has also shown us that community work can be considered to be part of a legitimation process which supports capitalism and creates the impression that community work can bring benefits to localities and groups rather than recognizing it is supporting a system based on exploitation.

An example of radical and socialist theory and its application to community work

Discussion in previous chapters has indicated that the British Community Development Projects of the late 1960s and the 1970s were the clearest example of the radical and socialist approaches to community work. Rejecting their conservative origins as determined by the Home Office, the Community Development Projects (CDPs) developed a Marxist structuralist analysis of social deprivation and argued that community work could function as a mechanism for social control. The CDPs' contribution to the development of community work theory has been much debated, with Thomas (1983) criticizing their 'doctrinaire style' and continuous devaluation of neighbourhood work which, he argues, alienated practitioners and inhibited open discussion. On the other hand, Waddington (1983), Craig et al. (2011) and Popple (2011) argue that the CDPs filled an ideological and theoretical vacuum, bringing a necessary coherence to community work. At the theoretical level, there is little doubt that the CDP offered a significant break with earlier traditions, and that their analysis has had a major impact not only upon community work but also within the arenas of social policy and local and central government. The strength of their arguments, Henderson (1983: 7) suggests, lay in the quality of their analysis which was grounded in careful local investigation and the reality of working-class experience, and their 'insistence on social class as the fundamental tool for understanding the areas where many community workers were employed'.

In relation to practice, it is harder to determine the influence of the CDPs. The problem, Waddington (1983: 42) suggests, lies partly in the fact that 'many community workers have found it difficult to operationalise or apply [radical] theory to their own practice, partly because the material produced by the Community Development Projects has tended to be longer on analysis than applications'.

According to Thomas (1983), the CDPs' attack on the value of neighbourhood work had a demoralizing effect on many workers at the time, undermining their faith and confidence in the potential of community work to effect social change. On a more positive note, their recognition of the importance of linking community and workplace struggles and the location of community work within a wider social analysis, which recognized the relationship between the economy and welfare provision, was invaluable. However, the CDPs have been criticized by feminists for being gender-blind, and by ethnic minority and anti-racist writers and activists as being 'colour'-blind. Both groups have criticized the CDPs, as well as the Left in general, for marginalizing their contributions and ignoring their experiences. Nevertheless, by rooting community work firmly in a structuralist analysis, the projects established the radical and socialist approach on a firm theoretical foundation. Socialist and radical theories, based upon a theory of class, are now less in evidence in community work than they were in the 1970s. There has, however, been an expansion in three significant strands of these theories that do not necessarily have class as their main focus but do contain a radical focus: (1) feminist theories; (2) the ethnic minority and the anti-racist critique; and (3) theories relating to environmentalism and the green movement.

Feminist theories

Feminism has a long history with the first 'wave' located in the eighteenth century with the works of the English writer, philosopher and advocate of women's rights, Mary Wollstonecroft (1757–1797). In the first part of the twentieth century we witnessed the rise of the women's suffrage movement in Britain and internationally which led to the enfranchisement of women which was discussed in Chapter 3. The second 'wave' of feminism in Britain came with the emergence of feminist theory, and in particular socialist feminist theory, during the late 1960s. This development was predated by the emergence of the male-dominated politically active grouping, the New Left, and the journal *New Left Review* which was launched in 1960. However, the developing feminist movement both in the UK and elsewhere led to a re-evaluation of male-influenced radical and socialist thinking. This developing analysis of women's subordinate position and the need for this to be addressed were later to influence community work theory and practice. This is discussed by, among others, Hanmer and Rose (1980) who point out that women, particularly those with young children, represent the key constituency for community work. The authors argue therefore that if community workers are to 'start where people are at', they have to take account of and relate to the experience of women's oppression.

From the mid-1990s and during the early part of the twenty-first century, third 'wave' (or 'new') feminism has gained ground as a counter to what are considered to be the new threats to women's bodies due to the impact of globalization, global terrorism, religious fundamentalism and genetic biotechnologies (Gillis et al. 2007). According to Krolloke and Sorensen (2006: 17), this 'new' feminism is 'characterized by local, national and transnational activism, in areas such as violence against women, trafficking, body surgery, self-mutilation, and the overall "pornification" of the media'.

At a theoretical level, there a number of different and often contested strands of feminism which have emerged since the establishment of 'second-wave' feminism in the late 1960s. Although this is not a comprehensive list of different approaches, the major strands of feminism include:

- *Liberal feminism* that focuses on the individual, and views the state as neutral. Liberal feminism is known for championing the case for improving women's position through increasing equal opportunities with men, in particular, in education, politics and employment. The writer and former British Conservative MP Louise Mench claims she is a feminist and from an analysis of her work, it would indicate that she is a liberal feminist.

- *Radical feminism* has as its core the analysis that society and the state are patriarchal and thus perpetuate gender inequalities, meaning that men remain in dominant and privileged positions and women are considered subordinate. In this paradigm male physical power is communicated through rape, sexual abuse and domestic violence (Bryson 1993). According to the Council of Europe (2006), it is believed that 12–15 per cent of all women have been in a relationship of domestic abuse after the age of 16.

- *Socialist and Marxist feminism* articulates the view that women's exploitation is due to capitalist economic relations which places them in a subordinate position to men. In particular, it presents the analysis that a patriarchal state and society encourage women to undertake unpaid work in the home and community while men derive the real material benefits from perpetuating this position. This feminist analysis focuses on class divisions while additionally stressing the particular disadvantages experienced by women.

- *Black and anti-racist feminism* has emerged as a response to the above theories which 'black' feminists argue tend to marginalize 'black' women and to render them invisible through its failure to account for their simultaneous oppressions by patriarchy, class and race. Further, the challenge to these failings lies in the questioning of categories and assumptions which are central to what is regarded as 'mainstream feminist thought' – specifically, white, middle-class feminist conceptualizations of patriarchy, the family and reproduction – which is rendered problematic when imposed upon the lives of black women (hooks 1997). 'Black' feminists within community work have struggled to put their theories into practice, often against a reaction both from other women and the state (Bhavnani 1982). 'Black' feminists also maintain that 'black' men similarly suffer from racism and on this central issue align themselves with them.
- *Postmodern feminism*, to quote Giddens and Sutton (2013: 658), rejects:

> the claim that there is a grand or overarching theory that can explain the position of women in society, or, indeed, that there is a universal category of 'woman' . . . instead, postmodernism encourages the acceptances of many different standpoints as equally valid. Rather than an essential core to womanhood, there are many individuals and groups, all of whom have very different experiences as heterosexuals, lesbians, black women, working-class women, and more.

One of the leading writers in the area of postmodern feminism is Judith Butler who argues that women's subordination is caused by a number of influences and her view is that there is no one solution to overcoming this factor. Butler (2006) challenges the category of 'woman' and the view that there is in fact a category termed 'feminine', arguing that this is a masculine construct. Like other postmodern feminist writers, Butler has sought to deconstruct male language and male views of the world. The argument continues that male is seen as normal and women as a deviation and there is a need therefore to reconstruct a view which is more fluid and open and reflects women's experiences.

We can see therefore there is a growing awareness among sociologists and other social scientists that class and gender inequality, racism, disability and other categories can be viewed as oppressions that are intersecting and they can be studied in a way that brings greater understanding of those experiencing these disadvantages. This view is well articulated by Collins (2000) and builds on the work of Ware (1991: xiv) who suggests the theoretical possibilities of 'finding a language that would express the links between race and gender, without prioritising and without oversimplifying . . . to work out ways of resisting one form of domination without being complicated in another'.

Declaring that the 'personal is political' (Millet 1969), the progressive elements of feminist theory and practice identified above can be seen to stress the political element in personal relationships and highlight the need to link home, workplace and the community. In more recent years, this message has been reiterated by the research undertaken by Walby (2011). Further, while emphasizing the importance of personal experience in developing links between women, feminist writers and workers have also stressed the centrality of personal experience and self-disclosure as a focus for work with women in the community (see, for example, Dominelli 2006; Ledwith and Springett 2010; Ledwith 2011). By highlighting the importance of personal experience, progressive feminist theory argues that while women may experience oppression differently and often individually, they share a common interest which inevitably influences the way they work and the issues they choose to work on. However, Smithies and Webster (1987) caution that common interests should not be used to advocate some utopian ideal of sisterhood. They argue that differences cannot and should not be minimalized or accommodated but instead could provide a starting point for the development of creative practical action for change. As Rowbotham (1979) has highlighted, it was in the context of the above that consciousness-raising groups emerged in Britain as a means of encouraging the reflection and action necessary for personal change and possible political transformation.

The ethnic minority and anti-racist community work critique

Just as socialist and radical feminist theory, 'black' and anti-racist feminist theory, and postmodern feminist theory have highlighted the need to reconstruct classical Marxist theory in the light of women's experience, so also the minority ethnic and anti-racist critique emphasizes the interrelation between 'race' and class, and to a lesser extent gender.

Since the publication of the first edition of *Analysing Community Work* in 1995, conceptualizing 'black' identity has undergone a major re-think. At the time when the first edition was written, the term 'black' was used in British society to refer to African, Caribbean and South Asian communities. Using this term also gave a political message that all 'black people' experienced racism and discrimination in a predominantly white country. However, as the late sociologist and cultural theorist Stuart Hall has argued, while using the term 'black' was politically useful during the early stages of post-war immigration (and a far more preferable term to that of 'coloured'), it was a 'necessary fiction' which tended to counter the racist line that 'white is good, black is bad' (Procter 2004: 123). The term 'black' was therefore in effect a social construction. What Hall proposes is a move from the umbrella term of 'black' to a position that considers the significant and at times contradictory complexities of 'race' and ethnicity. Hall terms these 'new ethnicities', which reflects the differences in and between diverse groups and enables those who reside in them to feel more comfortable with their chosen identity and to enjoy greater opportunities to express their voice (Hall 2006). This approach which rejects tightly drawn constructions of 'race' and ethnicity has much in common with postmodern thinking that celebrates the increasing changing nature and diversity of relationships and is critical of the universalizing aspects of Western philosophy and questions the view that there is a 'grand narrative' that guides the development of society. In line with Stuart Hall's view, the term ethnic minority groups is used here and which refers to those who have experienced racism by those in the 'majority'.

What is central in this critique is the view that Western capitalism is built on the foundations of slavery and imperialism from which it derived its wealth and power. The critique argues that this domination is perpetuated in the developing world through trade, aid and foreign debt. Further, that in Britain, state policy has operated as a repressive force on ethnic minority groups, particularly in relation to immigration policy and law and order policy. On a broader scale, there is recognition in the critical social sciences that racism operates at a personal and an institutional level as a material and ideological force permeating major institutions in society. For example, Graef (1989) found that police were 'actively hostile to all minority groups' while the public inquiry that commenced in 1998 into the 1993 racist murder of the black teenager Stephen Lawrence in south-east London concluded that the Metropolitan Police Service was 'institutionally racist' (Macpherson 1999). Further, people from ethnic minority groups are also more likely than whites to experience discrimination in the labour market (Hills et al. 2010) and in the housing market (Law 2010). Finally, Williams (1991) demonstrates the racist nature of the administration of welfare benefits and services and how black people's labour and resources were essential in creating the British welfare state.

In relation to community work, there have been two constant themes in the ethnic minority and anti-racist critique. One has been the resistance to racism, which Ohri et al. (1982) point out remains the primary issue for the ethnic minority community, and one which community work must address if it is to remain relevant to the needs and concerns of these groups. The other major theme has been the opportunities that community work has provided to different groups to encourage cultural formations in their own right. So we can see that in a highly complex and interwoven system of cultural overlap, people from ethnic minority groups have sustained and generated cultures and formations that not only react to discrimination and inequality but also create processes that have an identity and vitality of their own, independent of hostility from the dominant group.

Environmentalism and the green movement critique

In the last 20 years or more and since the publication of the first edition of *Analysing Community Work* there has been increasing international concern for environmental conservation and the need to restrict environmental damage caused mainly by intensified consumerism in developed economies. What were once seen as marginal ideas and practices related to protecting the environment are now considered to be mainstream, and globally we are more aware of the impact of global warming, overpopulation, air and water pollution, resource depletion, food shortages, GM crops, increasing consumerism, and the problems associated with the production of different forms of energy, including nuclear power and shale gas. While these major global complex issues can leave individuals feeling powerless to do very little to balance out these negative features, there have emerged a number of groups and movements both locally and internationally, that provide platforms for people to express their concern and to engage in social and community action.

Importantly too, theoretical perspectives have developed that reflect the need to create a society that has affordable, renewable and resilient energy sources; energy-efficient homes and workplaces; reliable, efficient and cheap public transport; dependable and convenient local food networks; and co-operative, diverse and resilient local economies built on sustainable growth (Woodin and Lucas 2004). These green alternatives to economic globalization are rooted in social and community action and are similar to the different perspectives discussed above in this chapter in that environmentalism is both a theoretical position and an ideology for action.

While there are a number of national and international pressure groups like Greenpeace and Friends of the Earth campaigning for significant changes in the way we consume and arguing for simpler ways of living, at a local community level there are numerous examples of people working together to address the negative impact of environmental degradation.

One movement that has been engaged in tackling the enormous environmental issues that presently face us is the Transition movement which unashamedly states it 'is a social experiment on a massive scale' (Hopkins 2011: 16). Although it started in the UK, its practical projects are found globally, including groups in Brazil, Germany, Japan, New Zealand and the USA. The work by Hopkins and others is based on the premise that 'If we wait for the government, it'll be too little, too late. If we act as individuals, it'll be too little. But if we act as communities, it might just be enough, just in time' (Hopkins 2011: 16). The main thrust of the Transition movement is centred on offering communities practical guidance and vision founded on community-based projects that value and encourage co-operation, creativity and the building of resilience. More information on the Transition movement can be found at: www.transitionnetwork.org

Evaluating community work theories

We have noted that though there is no one community work theory, the activity has been influenced by a number of macro-theories. Since the mid-1970s, community work advocates of these macro-theories have not enjoyed the smoothest of relationships, mainly because the advocates of socialist, radical, feminist theories, the ethnic minority and anti-racist critique, and the environmentalism and green movement critique which have shared critical perspectives, have been at variance with advocates of the pluralist theories. During the early 1970s, the socialist and radical theories of social, political and economic change came to challenge the dominant pluralist theories, leading to what one writer describes as a 'problematic discourse' between the main approaches to community work (Twelvetrees 2008).

It has been argued here that pluralist theories have resulted in the establishment of acceptable practice methods in order to handle state-defined prevailing social problems experienced in communities. This then assists in the efficiency and profitability of a social-democratic/neo-liberal market economy. The chosen form of social intervention is based on technical skills which can be at the expense of a critical appreciation of a changing social, economic and political world, or a commitment to being part of a significant change within society. We have noted that by concentrating on the marginal gains possible, pluralist community work theory can fail to make effective theoretical and practical connections between individuals' experience and the changing nature of society. Clearly pluralist theory involves value judgements, and though pluralist community work theories have never claimed to be value-free, we should be aware that its theories and practice values are not exposed fully, and therefore result in an aura of neutrality and objectivity. Another criticism of pluralist community work theory is that because of its key focus on the neighbourhood, it fails to connect sufficiently with the production and reproduction of inequalities in the wider society, which result in problems for localities.

Pluralist theories also emphasize the view that collective, social and institutionalized policies can stem only from government action or from the work of major community work agencies. This can omit a full appreciation of the unpaid army of people (usually women) who are engaged in, and have developed, community work practice. Pluralist community work theory tends to reflect the view that producing evidence on social problems will prompt a social conscience response. Its empiricist emphasis on the collection of 'facts', rather than on theory-building, gives credence to the view that piecemeal reform and intervention are possible and can be quantified or measured.

A further criticism of the pluralist community work theories is that community work tends to placate rather than liberate the individuals and groups that come within its orbit. It is something that is 'done to' rather than determined by a community. In this paradigm, community work is viewed as a professional and arguably elitist activity, undertaken by paid workers on behalf of agencies rather than by those living in a particular community. The reference group is the employing agency, not the community. Meanwhile pluralist community work theories often promote the concept of self-help and self-reliance, a concept that appeals to a wide political spectrum. Among those who favour this concept are those who believe in a centre right approach to social problems as well as those holding an anarchist, anti-statist view. The purpose of self-help here, however, is not to liberate a community, but to marshal 'community energies to replace public services rather than complement them' (Taylor 1992: 18).

On a more positive note, the pluralist approach has offered community work a range of practice theories and practical 'how-to-do-it' guidelines which are useful to practitioners of most ideological positions working in a wide range of statutory and voluntary bodies. In this way community work has come to influence other forms of practice in the public service, including social work, public health and education.

Community work theories which have evolved from classical Marxist theories, associated in practice with the class-orientated community action of the CDPs, have come to challenge the pluralist community work theories. These analyses have influenced not only the type of constituent groups worked with, but also the form of working and the values and principles that shape the community work being undertaken. These developments in community work theory have been underpinned and influenced by the growing macro-theoretical work that offers critical explanations about social phenomena.

The socialist community work theories provide an analysis of society which is a mixture of idealism and materialism. The idealism derives from the Fabian socialist tradition which, as we noted earlier, believes that it is possible to achieve change through rational discourse, the fostering of collective values and moral persuasion. This idealism is evident, for instance, in the belief that it is possible to prevent sexism or racism by educating people to act and think differently. Fabian socialism has been criticized by a number of writers, including Williams, who argues that it 'fails to recognize the bearing that society itself has on the creation and sustenance of ideas' (Williams 1991: 22).

This leads one to consider the notion of materialism. Marxists have demonstrated that ideas are inextricably linked to daily life. According to such theorists, ideas are shaped around the conflicts of interests between capital and labour, leading to struggle and change. In this paradigm, capital accommodates change and conflict. One of the arguments made of material Marxism is that it fails to fully recognize the resistance that comes from the grassroots and the potential for change that can come through resistance to an all-powerful hegemony. It is this materialist view that has been criticized by others on the Left who perceive the possibilities for change.

The main criticism that can be levelled at the radical and socialist theories is that practice by itself cannot change society. Socialism is both a political doctrine and a political movement containing a view of human action and a vision of human potential that are in essence internationalist or universal. 'Left' radicalism, on the other hand, offers a far-reaching critique of society that questions the very nature of the social, political and economic forces within society but does not offer a comprehensive and workable view of a future society. Both radical and socialist theories can lead to action in a whole range of fields, community work being one small segment. In order to achieve socialist goals, for instance, change has to be enacted at every level of society. Community workers, however, work with a numerically small and relatively powerless section of the population, and though practitioners influenced by socialist theories may attempt to 'prefigure' a more just and equal society, they will not alone achieve large-scale change. On a wider level, we have noted that the 'fall of socialism' in Eastern Europe and the former Union of Soviet Socialist Republics has led to questions of whether a Marxist material-ist position can successfully be put in place.

Feminist theories, the ethnic minority and anti-racist critique, and the environmentalism and green movement critique have, on the other hand, demonstrated that groups can, through collective action, successfully attempt to overcome problems facing them. Feminism, both as a socio-political theory and as a social movement, has, for instance, reconstructed perspectives in many different areas of life. Together, feminist theories, the ethnic minority and anti-racist critique, and the environmentalism and the green movement critique have implications for community work theory that do not rely on either localized analysis or materialist perspectives. In particular, the green critique and its application have much to offer contemporary community work as it has made recognizable attempts to link theories that analyse the impact of globalization and neo-liberalism with the possibilities of practice at the local level. In Chapter 6 we will consider how these developing themes can make for a more effective community work theory.

Question

1   What theory fits most comfortably with your view of the world? Consider the positive and negative aspects of the theory and its possible application to the practice of community work.

---

6 Community work theories for the twenty-first century

Introduction

In the previous chapter we reviewed the main theories that have informed community work, highlighting their different strengths and weaknesses. We have noted that while the pluralist theory has historically informed much of the dominant mode of community work in the UK and elsewhere, and its advocates have produced valuable how-to-do community work guides, it is the more critical perspectives that offer a new and progressive way forward for the activity. These critical perspectives are essential if we are to make connections between the wider forces of globalization, neo-liberalism and the resultant growing inequality, all of which are proving exceptionally challenging for communities and neighbourhoods in the twenty-first century.

This chapter will examine the role of community work in this broader setting and consider how we can use the writings of a number of progressive critical social theorists to enhance community work theory and practice. However, let us first remind ourselves of the context in which community work is located in the twenty-first century.

In Chapter 1 we considered the powerful forces of globalization and neo-liberalism and the resultant increasing inequality between and within nation states. Perhaps the foremost instrument of the massive economic and social change of the last 10 years that has developed and fed into these three factors has been the explosion in global communications with the development and spread of fibre-optic cables, together with telecommunication satellites that carry vast amounts of information that is often sent cheaply to destinations around the world in seconds. While this communication has increased information flows which have changed the economic context in which profit is made, we are also aware, as noted in Chapter 4, how contemporary social movements and networks have evolved and have been energized by the use of social media. These developments have enabled individuals and groups to communicate with each other in order to create an oppositional space against the negative impact of globalization and neo-liberalism. While there are concerns that the use of the internet and mobile technology will accelerate a global culture and in doing so diminish traditional cultures, it can also be argued that this has fashioned an important platform for sustaining and advancing democracy and participation which will counter the increasing individualism that capitalist relations depend upon for their sustainability.

These developments have implications for community work theories as we are now witnessing and participating in developments which are changing and will continue to change the world that we inhabit. In this context, therefore, it is opportune to first re-examine the work of the Italian social theorist, Antonio Gramsci (1891–1937), whose writings offer an understanding of the role that state workers such as community workers can play in assisting communities in uncertain times. These ideas were first developed in an article in a previously published community work volume (Popple 1994) and in the first edition of *Analysing Community Work*. Since then a number of community work commentators, including Ledwith (2011), and Beck and Purcell (2013) have made valuable contributions to our understanding of the value of Gramsci's theories.

After considering the concepts shaped by Gramsci, we will reflect on the implications of the work of the educator and philosopher, Paulo Freire (1921–97). Freire criticizes the 'banking' model of education which he claims fails to encourage the real development of individuals and communities. In its place he advocates critical pedagogy which similarly has much to offer community work.

Finally, we examine the contributions from a number of social theorists whose ideas resonate with the challenge facing community work in the twenty-first century. We conclude the chapter by linking some of the key themes offered by these writers, reflections on the role of social movements and new social movements, and then consider the implications for community work.

The theories of Antonio Gramsci: their contribution to community work theory

When Karl Marx produced his economic, political and social theories towards the end of the nineteenth century, they appeared to offer a clear vision of societal change by detailing what he considered would be the inevitable succession of the bourgeoisie by the proletariat. However, the increasing complexity of capitalist relations and changing social life in the twentieth and the twenty-first centuries has denied Marx's vision. What Marx failed to predict was the dominant or elite classes making willing and sometimes unwilling concessions to the subordinate classes and groups in order to maintain their privileged exclusive position and to ensure the successful continuation of profit for themselves and their dependants.

Writing after Marx and recognizing the inadequacies of his economic deterministic vision, the Italian social theorist, Antonio Gramsci instead focuses on key aspects of Marx's Hegelian, humanistic theory to reconceptualize the moral, philosophical and political spheres of social life. In doing so, Gramsci has provided us with an expanded vision of politics, one that rejects the concept of politics as solely being about electoral and narrow party politics, or the occupancy of state power. Instead Gramsci perceives politics as a struggle for moral and intellectual leadership. To quote Hall (1988: 169):

> Where Gramsci departs from classical versions of Marxism is that he does not think that politics is an arena which simply rejects already unified collective political identities, already constituted forms of struggle. Politics for him is not a dependent sphere. It is where forces and relations, in the economy, in society, in culture, have to be actively worked on to produce particular forms of domination. This is the production of politics – politics as a production. This conception of politics is fundamentally open-ended.

This view is one which assists us in our development of a more enhanced community work theory applicable to the present times. One of the most positive aspects of Gramsci's work is its rejection of the rudimentary but arguably inspiring historical materialist analysis. This analysis was reflected in the writings of the Marxist Left and socialist groups during the 1960s and 1970s and was to have some influence on those engaged in the Community Development Projects as well as the radical and socialist community workers of the period that we discussed in Chapters 4 and 5. Instead, Gramsci's work provides us with an analysis of how groups and individuals can shape developments within society. Here his concepts of hegemony, ideology and intellectuals are the most relevant.

Gramsci (1971; 1975; 1977; 1978) discusses the notion that any ruling elite dominates subordinate classes and groups with a combination of force and consent. He argues that force is exercised through the armed forces, the police, the law courts and prisons, while consent is gained through the political, moral and intellectual leadership within civil society. This domination is maintained by a process of hegemony which has been described as

> the relation between classes and other social forces. A hegemonic class, or part of a class, is one which gains the consent of other classes and social forces through creating and maintaining a system of alliance by means of political struggle.

> (Simon 1982: 22)

Gramsci argues that civil society, which has been defined by Gramscians as consisting of organizations such as political parties, trade unions, churches and cultural, charitable and community groups, is central in sustaining the hegemony. According to Gramscians, civil society is the sphere where popular-democratic struggles are grouped together – 'race', gender, age, community, ethnicity, nation, and so forth – and it is here that the struggle for hegemony takes place. These struggles have been identified as social movements, and we will return to them later in the chapter.

To achieve an effective hegemony, Gramsci argued, there must be a number of beliefs or ideas which are generally accepted by all but which serve to justify the interests of the dominant groups. These images, concepts and ideas which 'make sense' of everyday experiences are collectively known as an 'ideology'. Gramsci argues that ideology is the cement that keeps society together and any change in ideology has to be undertaken at the institutional level. However, Gramsci also argues that the subordinate classes or groups do not necessarily have the conceptual tools to comprehend the situation fully, or the means to formulate the radical alternatives to change the ideology or over-come the hegemonic forces. If change is to take place, Gramsci believes that 'external agents', in the guise of intellectuals, organizers and leaders, are necessary. Gramsci's definition of 'intellectuals' extends beyond the tradition-ally held notion of thinkers, philosophers, artists, journalists and writers, to include organizers such as civil servants and political leaders who are active in civil society, as well as engineers, managers and technicians who function in the production sphere. Gramsci describes 'organic' intellectuals as those who have been created by a particular class and 'give it homogeneity and an awareness of its own function not only in the economic but also in the social and political fields' (Gramsci 1971: 5). These intellectuals are members of the class they represent. Thus, a dominant class creates its own intellectuals in the form of economists, civil servants, industrial managers, writers and media personnel who reflect and support the values of that class.

Returning to our consideration of community work, we can pose the question: are community workers 'organic' intellectuals? In reply, we can observe that most practitioners are employed in one way or another by the state and are therefore acting with particular instructions or authority, so that they could be considered to be a subordinate branch of the dominant 'organic' intel-lectuals. On the other hand, the fact that they can be at odds with the dominant ideology and are encouraging individuals and groups to articulate their own discourse means they do not fully agree with the dominant system. Therefore, it could be interpreted that community workers are strategic players in helping people make connections between their position and the need for change.

To help us understand and clarify the role of community workers in this paradigm, we can refer to Simon (1982), who argues that certain groups of workers are part of an important 'middle stratum' which has particular professional and corporate interests and traditions. Simon believes it is the specialized training provided in institutions such as colleges that separates the 'middle stratum' from the vast majority of workers.

> They have been constituted into a variety of 'middle strata' capable of playing a distinctive part in politics which can be very significant indeed. They are therefore a vital component of the broad alliance which has to be built up by the working class if it is to achieve a hege-monic role in society.
>
> (Simon 1982: 98)

Gramsci and Simon demonstrate, however, that members of this 'middle stratum' can hold traditional views and act as instruments of political stabil-ity. For instance, Gramsci is critical of the conservative role adopted by certain trade unions and their leaders in working within bourgeois demo-cracy. Similarly, he argues that the economic and political system does not represent the non-elite and consequently there is always the potential for social disintegration. These observations would indicate that community workers have a role in facilitating the response of the non-elite and a role in the changing of social circumstances.

Aspects of Gramsci's theories, then, offer us a workable framework for our examination of community work theory. His theories reject the notion of class agents as the sole bearers of change, and more importantly the concept of one hegemonic centre in society. Dominant groups maintain and reproduce their ascendancy through a complex web of ideological processes in an attempt to establish an agreed understanding of reality. This understanding of reality is intended to permeate our principles, social relationships and intellec-tual and moral positions. However, according to Gramscians, this understand-ing is never completely secure because our daily experiences of the world are frequently at odds with the view offered by bourgeois ideology. We can, there-fore, simultaneously hold different and apparently contradictory and incon-sistent interpretations of the world – one determined and shaped by the prevailing dominant ideology, and the other determined by our everyday experiences in communities which give us 'common-sense' knowledge. In this paradigm community workers are situated in a pivotal position in the civil society, for though they are employees of the state and are required to play a part in maintaining the social system, they are not necessarily in agreement with its ideology. Accordingly, community workers have opportunities to work alongside members of communities as they articulate their contradict-ory understanding of the world and their situation within it (see Figure 6.1). This theory also proposes that community work is concerned with moving from the terrain of ideas and discussion and into transforming action to change people's material situation.

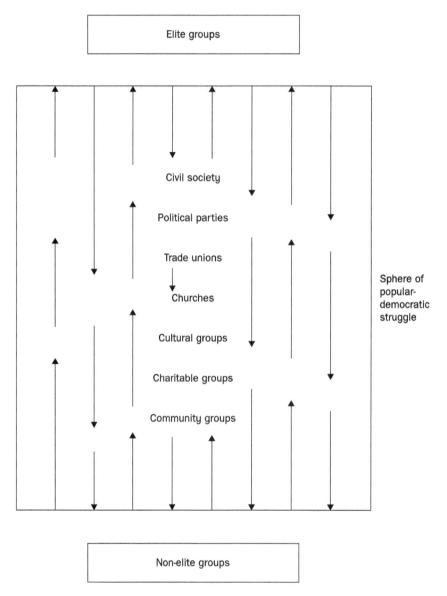

Figure 6.1 Hegemony and the sphere of popular-democratic struggle.

Freed from the boundaries of the economic Marxist determinist position, Gramsci's theoretical work allows us to develop concepts that enable us to locate community work within a site of resistance. These developing Gramscian concepts, the complementary analysis provided by a number of social theorists, and a consideration of the role of social movements and new social movements enable us to apply it to community work which we will consider later in this chapter.

Now that we have a valuable handle on how to understand hegemony in society and how it is possible to find oppositional space in order to work for change, we turn to the work of the Brazilian educator, Paulo Freire, whose main focus is the use of education for transformation and whose work was to challenge school-based interventions.

The theories of Paulo Freire: their contribution to community work

Working with poverty-stricken South American communities during the 1960s, Paulo Freire found ways of developing approaches through which people can express their feelings and experiences and in doing so to regain their sense of humanity and then take action to change their circumstances. Freire argues that the dominant social relations create for many people a culture of silence that results in their oppressed negative and usually suppressed feelings about themselves. His educational approach, however, is aimed at changing this by showing how educators can work alongside those considered oppressed in order that they can reflect on their experiences and question what was previously taken for granted.

Freire therefore proposes an educational process which rejects the traditional hierarchical 'banking' system, where knowledge is considered to be a commodity accumulated in order to gain access to positions of power and privilege. In his seminal work, *Pedagogy of the Oppressed* (1970), Freire argues that the way in which the majority of education is delivered means that students become receiving objects. He argues that the students' ideas and action are in effect measured and contained, leading them to adjust to the world around them and inhibiting their creative tendencies.

Education for Freire is a political act and he developed a philosophy and practice termed 'education for liberation' whereby learners and teachers engage in a process in which abstract and concrete knowledge, together with experience, are integrated into *praxis* (which can be defined as action intended to alter the material and social world). The fundamental features of this praxis are critical thinking and dialogue (as opposed to discussion) which seek to challenge conventional explanations of everyday life, while at the same time considering the action necessary for the transformation of oppressive conditions.

The extensive work of Freire (1970; 1972; 1976; 1985) centres on the concept of 'conscientization', otherwise known as politicization and political action. According to Freire, before people can engage in action for change, they have first to reflect upon their present situation. However, the nature of ideological domination means that subordinate groups accept, and frequently collude with, the reproduction of a society's inequalities and the explanations and justifications offered for the status, power and privilege of their oppressors: an idea similar to notions developed by Gramsci. Overcoming this false ideology means overcoming people's pessimistic and fatalistic thinking. Freire understood this was not an easy task, but his great optimism and purpose have led to educators around the world taking up the challenge.

Freire argues that educators have to work on the wide range of experiences brought by oppressed people. The educational process entails providing opportunities for people to validate their experiences, culture, dreams, values and histories, while recognizing that such expressions carry both the seeds of radical change and the burden of oppression. Freire's position coincides with that held by many community workers that it is necessary to start from a person's own understanding. According to Freire, the skill is to work with people by a 'problematizing' approach rather than a 'problem-solving' stance as advocated in the 'banking' system of education. 'Problem-solving' involves an expert being distant from a person's reality while engaging in an analysis that efficiently resolves difficulties before dictating a strategy or policy. Freire believes that this reduces human experience and difficulties to that which can be 'treated'. 'Problematizing', however, means immersing oneself in the struggle of disadvantaged communities and engaging in the task 'of codifying total reality into symbols which can generate critical consciousness' (Freire 1976: ix).

According to Freire, this empowers people to begin to alter their social relations which are undertaken by a process of critical reflection and action followed by further critical reflection and action, and so on. This, he argues, creates conditions for the development of genuine theory and collective action because both are rooted in a historical and cultural reality. However, Freire believes that theory and practice are not conflated into one another. Instead, there needs to be distance between the two: 'Theory does not dictate practice; rather, it serves to hold practice at arm's length in order to mediate and critically comprehend the type of praxis needed within a specific setting at a particular time in history' (Freire 1985: xxiii).

Allman (1987) claims that Freire's ideas have begun to permeate liberal education in the United Kingdom but because of the structure and underlying ideology of the present system, they are likely to be used only selectively. Further, Allman (1987: 214) writes that Freire's ideas have been distorted and devalued in the 'futile attempt to incorporate "radical" technique in the "liberal" agenda'. Taking note of these criticisms, we can see that Freire's work, together with the writings of Gramsci, has implications for the theory and practice of community work.

Other contributions to community work theory-building

Gramsci and Freire are not the only thinkers and activists who can make a contribution to an enhanced community work theory that resonates with the challenges we now face. There are a number others whose work can be drawn on individually and collectively to sharpen our understanding of the link between ideas and action. These writers are Saul Alinsky, Manuel Castells, Michel Foucault, bell hooks, Steven Lukes and Amartya Sen and are listed and commented on here alphabetically.

Saul Alinsky

As we noted in Chapter 3, Saul Alinsky (1902–72) was a controversial community organizer operating in Chicago particularly during the 1930s and whose seminal work for grass-root organizing, *Rules for Radicals* (1971), was to have a major impact on methods which help to inform how best to achieve success in campaigns. The 'rules' Alinsky developed were based on successes he had with a number of campaigns with those living in economically poor 'ghettos' and wanting to confront the privileges of the rich and powerful. Alinsky and his many followers worked in a unified manner with people to build grass-root People's Organizations that took on power brokers such as major local employers and public bodies. Alinsky's strategy was to work to restore dignity to those living in poor areas by helping them to organize in order to fight racism, discrimination and poverty. His tactics were undoubtedly confrontational and oppositional but they were also non-violent, creative and inventive; the very same tactics many would argue that are needed in contemporary times.

In Chapter 3 we discussed Alinsky's view that people are primarily motivated by self-interest. As we commented, and quoting Beck and Purcell (2013), this does not mean that people are individually motivated for private gain. Rather that a group of people who share the same self-interest (say, to protect their local community which is under threat) can work effectively together as they are driven by something that is beyond the power of one person.

The 12 'rules' Alinsky identifies for pressurizing major bodies to take account of the needs and wants of neighbourhood residents are as powerful now as when written. They provide anyone wanting to engage in improving neighbourhood life with guidelines that are based on starting from people's expressed concern for change. One of his 'rules' states that power is not only what you have, but what an opponent thinks you have. He suggests if your organization is small, you shouldn't reveal the number of people you have but rather make a 'noise' so that it appears you have more people than others think you have. Alinsky also writes that community workers should make their opponents live up to their own 'rules': 'You can kill them with this, for they can no more obey their own rules than the Christian church can live up to Christianity' (Alinsky 1971: 128).

There is no doubt that Alinsky's ideas and his 'rules', which he emphasizes must be understood as fluid and responsive, have a great deal of significance in contemporary community work thinking as his analysis and practice are based on an analysis of power and how to confront it. Power is a theme studied closely by Michel Foucault and Steven Lukes, both of whom we consider later in the chapter.

Manuel Castells

The Spanish sociologist, Manuel Castells (1942–) has researched extensively on a number of issues pertinent to community life and in particular he has made valuable contributions to urban sociology, social movements, the information society, and globalization.

Castells argues that urban problems are a direct result of the relationship between capitalism and urbanism. He views the production process as being at the heart of capitalism, with the city or communities as the site of the process of the reproduction of labour. Castells contends that the reproduction of labour power has gradually become mediated through collective rather than individual means which have brought with them a series of contradictions which may, in time, cause a 'revolutionary rupture' in society. According to Castells, the major contradiction lies in the economic needs of capital and the need to reproduce labour. Private capital by itself cannot provide for the state's citizens and has therefore to intervene on a large scale in the area of housing, health care, education, public transport, and so on. Castell termed the concept 'collective consumption' and argued it is in this area that there are possibilities to engage in struggles to improve community life. He comments that: '[Capitalism] globalizes and politicizes all the problems in making their collective treatment more necessary and visible but at the same time in making their confrontation by the individual more difficult' (Castells 1975: 190). This contradiction paves the way for the 'dialectic between the state apparatus, and urban social movements' (Castells 1977: 463).

Castells argues that if people want to achieve change, they need to form social movements or organizations with the aim of benefiting from these contradictions, stating that these organizations will frequently cut across class, gender, and ethnic divides as a combination of groups and classes will demand the same change.

Castells' more recent work focuses on the information society and globalization. In Chapter 4 we noted one of Castells' current contributions (Castells 2012) in which he explores new forms of social movements and protests groups that are using communication networks such as the internet, mobile phones and wireless communication in order to organize and publicize their causes. Castells argues that these new forms of organization and the tactics they deploy are beyond classic political party infrastructures and provide us with a further understanding of our changing social and political world, not only in Arab countries, Spain and the USA, to which he gives most attention but also in other countries. His argument is that the internet and other forms of communication have been used by protestors to counter the effects of oppression and injustice and provide us with different ways of engaging in social change and political democracy.

A prolific writer and one of the world's most cited social science academics, he has also produced a ground-breaking trilogy of texts in *The Information Age: Economy, Society and Culture* (Castells, 2000a; 2000b; 2004). In this trilogy Castells argues that network organizations are replacing vertically integrated hierarchies as the dominant form of organization. This enables people to move between different landscapes and work in different ways, some of which are oppositional and provide social and community activists with space to inter-relate and organize. Groups such as the protest groups UK Uncut is an example of such an organization. UK Uncut is a network of protest groups which arose in response to the reports in 2010 that Vodafone was avoiding paying UK tax and has since engaged through its vertical hierarchy in other campaigns against large retail groups such as Boots, Fortnum and Mason, and Starbucks, and banks such as HSBC, RBS and Barclays, see: www.ukuncut.org.uk/ (accessed 24 February 2014).

Michel Foucault

Probably one of the most controversial and at times puzzling to understand of all social theorists of recent times is the French philosopher, social theorist and literary critic, Michel Foucault (1926–84), whose work overlaps with a number of different disciplines. Foucault argues that these disciplines are by their nature conditional and historical. One of the key ideas that Foucault offers us is an exposition of power, contending that power is everywhere rather than located in the property of one person or class. For Foucault, power is a relation.

A social activist at different times during his life, Foucault argues that power operates *through* people rather than *on* people. Using the example of the modern prison system, he argues that power in such institutions is coercive and dissipated and operates in a manner that appears unobtrusive, relatively humane and painless, which is very different from the prisons of the past which were physically brutal, inhuman and places of torture and capital punishment. However, Foucault (1977) states that both forms of prisons (old and modern) regulate, discipline and punish. One is a based on imprisoning and torturing the body. The other is focused on punishing the soul.

Foucault then uses this analogy to examine society and argues that in modern times technologies of surveillance are used to control and dominate people. He argues that for this to happen, subjects must to be willing and compliant (Foucault 1980). From a reading of Foucault's work, the message for community work theory is that power is actually a form of power struggle and members of the dominant group or elites are focused on disciplining subjects to keep them docile and accepting, so that society can be managed in an orderly manner. In order for this to happen, everyone needs to have a function and role that is agreed. For example, in a school there is usually a head teacher, heads of subjects, class teachers and teaching assistants, all located in a hierarchy and all can claim authority over the school students. These roles enable surveillance to take place so that people's behaviour is regulated and controlled and discipline is exercised. Foucault argues that the exercise of this power is based primarily upon knowledge, which, as we have seen, involves collating information on people's activities. This knowledge then further reinforces exercises of power.

Importantly Foucault's analysis of surveillance and power provides us with an understanding of new managerialism which we discussed in Chapter 1 and which is a feature of neo-liberalism. In both the private and public sectors, this management style has been introduced through electronic monitoring instruments, including the sharing of electronic diaries (which, if they are located on employer-provided tablets or laptops, can be tracked by employers); cameras and CCTV recording; enforcing individual appraisals, focused on department and corporate goals, where workers are required to demonstrate key performance indicators; the encouragement and rewarding of authoritarian management styles; and the imposition of open plan offices enabling managers to deploy visual surveillance of workers. All these surveillance mechanisms intrude on personal privacy and individual trust and challenge the basis of a viable public life that maintains democratic values and practices.

In relation to community work, this has minimized opportunities for creating oppositional space with workers required to accept these dominant forms of oppressive management. However, Foucault argues that there is always the possibility of resistance, no matter how powerful and oppressive the system is, as power and resistance always co-exist. An excellent example of power and resistance but on a different level and in the theatre of war is the compelling and poignant account by an ex-British soldier Eric Lomax (2005) of his experience as a prisoner of the Japanese during the Second World War. Although Lomax and his colleagues were routinely tortured and brutally treated by their captors, they discovered a number of ways in which to resist their captors in order to survive and bring them some sense of humanity and hope despite their appalling treatment.

bell hooks

A black American feminist theorist and social activist, *bell hooks* (1952–) is the nom de plume for Gloria Jean Watkins. The name originates from hooks honouring both her maternal grandmother, who had the name Bell Hooks, and her mother. However, hooks decided not to capitalize her adopted name so as to distinguish herself from her grandmother while establishing for herself a 'separate voice' from her given and family names.

A prolific writer and media commentator, bell hooks has published books and journal articles covering many areas, including gender, 'race', history, art and the significance of the mass media for culture. Some of these publications are scholarly texts while others are more popular mainstream work, including films. A Buddhist, her unique style draws on a range of other scholars and activists, including James Baldwin, and the civil rights leaders Martin Luther King Jr. and Malcolm X, as well as drawing inspiration from Paulo Freire, the German-American psychologist Erich Fromm and the Vietnamese Buddhist monk Thicht Nhat Hanh.

Presently Distinguished Professor of English at City College, New York, hooks is known principally for her postmodern approach to writing, with her style moving between different forms, tones and styles in order to best project her ideas and feelings. A key focus of her work is the interconnectivity of 'race', capitalism and gender. This approach was laid out in her first major work (hooks 1981), which proved ground-breaking in trying to capture the complex links between different oppressions. Through a feminist analysis, hooks examines the complex relations between various forms of oppression and in particular the impact of sexism on black women during slavery, including the historic devaluing of black women, of black male sexism, of racism within the women's movement, and black women's involvement with feminism. In this seminal work, hooks offers a powerful critique of the way that many women have appropriated feminism for their own ends and to further their own careers. hooks argues that many of these women (usually white women) have been leading members of the feminist movement. She maintains that a more appropriate term is 'feminist' rather than 'feminism', which means everyone, both female and male, should be encouraged to liberate themselves from sexist roles and oppression.

However, it is in the area of education for liberation that hooks provides us with valuable material for community work theory. Influenced by the work of Freire, she argues that his ideas helped her affirm her 'right as a subject in resistance to define reality' (1994: 53). In the same book she contends that, similar to the views of Freire, she believes classrooms can be oppressive places in which through the traditional 'banking' system people can be fashioned into automatons as they are not exposed to critical thinking. Instead hooks maintains that classrooms and education generally can be used in ways which generate more creative, liberated and engaged people. Her view is that to achieve a more transformative position with people in an education setting, it is critical to make a firm commitment to work from a 'lived understanding' of people's lives in place of what hooks calls the distortion of a 'bourgeois lens' (hooks 1993: 151).

In her analysis of the writings of Freire, hook argues she has intertwined the South American educator's pedagogy and her own feminist pedagogy which has been informed by her experience of racism, to enlighten her teaching and writing (hooks 1993: 150). This is a particularly significant point as Freire's analysis has been challenged by some feminists, including hooks, as failing to satisfactorily acknowledge the gendered nature of oppression and disadvantage.

Steven Lukes

The British political and social theorist Steven Lukes (1941–) has contributed to our understanding of power through his classic text, *Power: A Radical View*, which was updated from its first edition to include two major new essays. This seminal text, published in 2005, presents what he terms as a 'three-dimensional view' of power.

Lukes takes issue with the Foucauldian idea that power is present in all social relations in equal measure. Instead in his exploration of the third dimension of power Lukes contends that the powerless internalize their position and take on the roles of worker and consumer. This dimension of power arises in the apparent absence of conflict and grievances and may involve the powerless consuming material goods, or absorbing and colluding with certain ideologies so accepting the power structure as the 'natural order of things'. According to Lukes, the real needs and the 'true interests' of the dominated are obscured and he introduces the concept of 'false consciousness' where the dominated have been misled through forces such as disinformation and censorship.

The sociological study by Lukes of power makes a valuable contribution to our understanding of this key concept and though his work could be interpreted as generally a pessimistic one, it can be placed alongside our discussion of power as articulated by Gramsci and Freire.

Amartya Sen

Amartya Sen (1933–) is an Indian economist and a Nobel Laureate who has made valuable contributions to our understanding of welfare economics and economic and social justice. Of Sen's many theories, there are two specific observations that can contribute to our aspiration to enhance community work theory.

The first relates to global inequality. Sen (2001) argues that the crude economic measures used to understand global inequality are inadequate. Instead Sen claims that there is a need to link economics with a political philosophy that makes a connection between material improvements and political and societal participation, and which advances human rights and demands changes in key institutions.

Sen maintains that theories of development have to recognize that 'development' is ultimately a matter of human freedom. He argues that people living in poverty, social deprivation, under political tyranny or cultural authoritarianism in the developing world are in effect imprisoned by these negative forces. He contends that governments and international organizations need to review their public policies from the perspective of freedom, and he maintains that institutions like political parties, the judiciary and the media can contribute to the development of enhancing individual and group freedom.

Sen's view is that we all want to lead a life of value. To achieve this, those who are imprisoned by 'unfreedoms' must be given the chance to enjoy the normal chances to live with sufficient income, to enjoy economic and educational opportunities, to benefit from good health and decent living standards, and all without being the victims of discrimination, repression and arbitrary justice. Sen argues that true economic improvement is that which benefits a cross-section of society (rather than a privileged elite), and where economic and social justice is fully conspicuous in a world that offers opportunities to increase the range of human choice.

We can see here the writings by Sen resonate with the same understanding that most in community work share; that the emphasis on the supremacy of economic goals, whether in the developed or developing world, is usually at the expense of the poor and to the benefit of the rich. One of the key values of community work is that of challenging economic and social injustice and offering alternative ways of living. Sen's evaluation of the need to bring 'humanity' rather than 'economics' to the forefront therefore provides us with a valuable analysis to assist the development of a progressive community work theory.

The second contribution Sen can make to community work theory lies in his challenge to the 'solitarist approach' which perceives a person's nationality, their religious adherence, and their cultural background to be their main form of identity. Instead Sen (2007: xii) argues that we all belong to a range of different groups and every day we move between different contexts and people view us in different ways. He presents this idea in the following manner:

> The same person can be, without any contradiction, an American citizen, of Caribbean origin, with African ancestry, a Christian, a liberal, a woman, a vegetarian, a long-distance runner, a historian, a schoolteacher, a novelist, a feminist, a heterosexual, a believer in gay

and lesbian rights, a theatre lover, an environmental activist, a tennis fan, a jazz musician, and someone who is deeply committed to the view that there are intelligent beings in outer space with whom it is extremely urgent to talk to (preferably in English). Each of these collectivities to all of which this person simultaneously belongs, gives her a particular identity. None of them can be taken to be the person's only identity or singular membership category.

Sen's view that people enjoy a plurality of individual identities is a valuable but problematic one for community work. As we saw above, Castells and Alinsky both recognize that the need to achieve certain goals for groups cuts across divides such as ethnicity, gender and class and can unite a diverse range of people in campaigns. In this case the individuals share the same identity and want to achieve the same objective. However, within that group there will be individuals who are disadvantaged because they are a member of an ethnic minority, or are disabled or are discriminated against because of their sexual orientation, or can be classified as being a member of all three groups. For these individuals, their identity as being part of a disadvantaged group could weigh heavily on them in their encounters with other group members.

The potential contribution of the study of social movements and new social movements to community work theory

In the section above we have presented the work of eight leading social theorists and social and community activists who in their different ways provide us with a more inclusive and critical approach to understanding community work and the theories that can be applied to the activity. The themes raised by the commentators are in a number of places linked to interventions by social movements and new social movements which can be described as collective attempts to further a common interest or goal outside the sphere of established institutions. As this chimes with an increasing number of campaigns at the local and neighbourhood level through what is usually called community action in the UK and elsewhere, it is appropriate for us to examine the nature of social movements and new social movements.

The theories relating to social movements and new social movements that are of particular help in our discussion of community work theory discuss the link of micro-interventions to macro-movements. As we can note, there are two sorts of movements. One is *social movements* which has been part of a popular dissent for over two hundred years (Tilly 2004) and focuses on a particular social or political issue. There are numerous examples of social movements in the last century, including the formation of the socialist and Communist Parties in Russia which led to the Russian Revolution of 1917; the non-violent, civil disobedience movements in India in the 1940s which was an element of the struggle for independence from the British; the American Civil Rights Movement of the 1960s which demanded total civil rights and full equality for all American citizens; and the Polish Solidarity movement in the late twentieth century that through a combination of labour and civil rights groups pressed for an end to a centralized economic and political system and the founding of social democracy.

In many ways *new social movements* are not unlike social movements except they are more recent in emergence and instead of focusing on material and economic gains, they are concentrated on issues relating to lifestyle, identity and culture. Examples include the Greens, the women's movement, the gay and lesbian rights movement and in more recent times the global anti-capitalist Occupy Movement. Unlike social movements where the membership is likely to be broad based, there is a view that those involved in new social movements are usually drawn from the middle classes.

New social movements usually comprise of a coalition of loosely knit groups that stand in oppositional alliance to a whole sphere of developments that are taking place in society, with some having the potential for greater radical change than others (Buechler 1999). Although these groups have national and even international profiles, they draw considerable strength from neighbourhood and urban-based activity that links them with each other through publications, conferences, rallies, meetings, demonstrations and civil disobedience.

One of the major themes of new social movements is 'act locally, think globally'. In the development of these movements it is possible to detect a strong concern among their members to avoid being subsumed by political ideologies, and to define their own goals, limits and forms of action. Of prime importance is the desire to organize around the mobilization of people within society, rather than to seize power, though, as we saw in elements of the Arab Spring uprisings, the goal was to remove groups and people with power and replace them with alternative groups and individuals.

Fundamentally both social movements and new social movements are a reaction to the failure of the major political parties to break out of conventional methods of organizing, as well as a response to a range of issues of a global and local concern that demand direct action. Such movements, it has been argued, are at the forefront of responding to problems as they collide with people's everyday experiences. They are not only engaged in challenging the activity of the state and civil society in a variety of areas, but also involved in proposing and initiating alternatives.

The women's movement has been particularly active in encouraging and developing alternative approaches to theory and practice in political organization. Women, who are frequently the cornerstone of many new social movement developments, have over many years made demands on such issues as equal pay, abortion and contraception, legal rights and protection against domestic violence, while offering a number of working theories and practices which challenge the culture of patriarchy. For example, as we discussed in Chapter 5, Rowbotham (1992) and other feminist writers argue for the need to bring together people's experience of organizing in order to replace the old forms of political structure which they believe fail to respond to grassroots demands.

There are a number of implications regarding the theories of social movements and new social movements that relate to community work theory. Many movements, and in particular new social movements, have come to challenge values at an individual and a societal level and their use of consciousness-raising and anti-discriminatory practice, and their participatory and non-hierarchical approaches to organizing, are a central feature and resonate with community work approaches. Similarly, the deconstruction and reconstruction of language – for instance, the use of 'gay' for 'homosexual', 'black' for 'negro', 'woman' for 'girl' – is part of a discourse that has its roots within the social movements.

As we discussed earlier in this chapter, both Freire and Foucault have highlighted the historical formation of cultural practices and discourses. For example, Freire's work highlights how people have been silenced or 'denied their voice' and stresses the importance of dialogue in the struggle of people who wish to become 'beings of self'. Foucault meanwhile, has drawn attention to discourse and practice. For Foucault, power is in our action not our heads. Fraser (1989: 25), discussing Foucault, claims he means that 'practices are more fundamental than belief systems when it comes to understanding the hold that power has on us'. According to Foucault, the acceptance of certain discourses comes to validate certain versions of the truth. The establishing of alternative discourses, like those that have emerged from the social movements and new social movements can, Foucault claims, help to break truth from the 'forms of hegemony' in which it operates.

What can community work theory gain from the literature relating to social movements and new social movements? First, it is important to state that, while there are views that new social movements are not necessarily 'new' and have been part of elements of social movements for many years, and new social movements are almost wholly left-wing, with there being little evidence of right-wing social movements or new social movements, these and other claims do not diminish the pivotal role both types of movements have had in modern life.

The key for us is whether such movements offer us lessons for community work. In some instances there are similarities, as there is the connection between localized neighbourhood demands and the need to take a more global view, which the social theorists we have discussed have highlighted. While it is possible to argue that community action is usually limited, small-scale reactions to problems and issues, there is in this arena the possibility of making connections between individuals' experiences and the nature of contemporary society. For example, over many years links have been made between the women's demands in neighbourhoods and the women's movement, and between the peace movement and the Greens. A central feature here is the cultural dimension of social action. Such action is both reactive and proactive as it attempts to develop new theories and practice. Community work, with its wealth of experience and skill in working in some of the poorest neighbourhoods, has, it would appear, the potential to feed into the debates surrounding social movements and new social movements.

The benefit for community work theory is an expanded understanding of the nature of macro-forces which shape and impinge upon individuals and communities. Similarly, an understanding of the literature and sociological theory relating to social movements and new social movements provides a broad background which could inform the practice of community work but can also be tempered by an awareness of the useful existing community work theory. We will return to consider these points in Chapter 10.

Conclusion

We noted in Chapter 5 that it is not possible to talk of a unified community work theory, but rather a number of macro-theories which have served to underpin and assist community workers, and explain and develop their work. Perhaps one salient reason for this lack of a clear theoretical base is the unique way in which community work responds to specific local conditions, making it difficult to provide examples of work that can be generalized.

In reviewing the established theories, we identified their strengths and weaknesses, concluding that the pluralist theories have failed to fully appreciate an important literature that offers community work a means of further theorizing and understanding its role and operation, while recognizing a wider remit.

In this chapter, we have drawn on the work of Gramsci, Freire, Alinsky, Castells, Foucault, hooks, Lukes and Sen, as well as considering developments in social movements and new social movements to demonstrate that communities can be one specific site in the resistance to different hegemonies. The community worker usually locates her/himself with the oppressed or subordinate groups and is therefore sometimes seen as politically radical. In order to challenge existing power structures, this radicalism may require a variety of theoretical perspectives to respond to a variety of social hegemonies. The lessons from the social theorists and social and community activists, and social and new movements, is that the background assumptions that operate in social relations can be challenged. This has implications for community work practice. First, this requires a flexible community work practice responsive to the local conditions in which the worker finds her/himself. The skills and settings for this practice are discussed in subsequent chapters. Second, while local task-orientated community work is progressing, wider developments, sometimes at a global level, are taking place. This needs to be recognized and appreciated if community work is to be more than the localized neighbourhood activity that is advocated by the pluralist theorists.

Questions

1 Consider the work of the social theorists presented here. Which of their theories most can help you in developing a theory and practice for community work?

2 Are there other social theorists whose work you consider to be of value in developing our understanding of community work? Who are these theorists and how does their work make a contribution to the activity of community work?

3 Consider one new social movement. What impact does it have at a local level? What role does it play in a broader context?

---

7 Community work models

Introduction

The previous chapters have provided us with a developing and critical understanding of community work. In Chapters 3 and 4 we discussed the emergence of British community work from its different roots and traditions up to the contemporary context, viewing it alongside a number of major changes in the economic, social and political fields, both nationally and internationally. In Chapter 5 we examined the various and often competing theories that inform community work, recognizing that there is no one theory that meets with universal agreement. In Chapter 6 we examined different complementary sociological theories and approaches together with a review of the influence of key thinkers, social movements and new social movements, all of which can be used to better understand and act on the challenges facing present-day community work.

Throughout this work our discussions have recognized that community work can be conceptualized around both theory and practice, and though they are inextricably linked, for our own purposes it is more productive initially to consider each of them separately. The focus of this chapter is to reflect upon the theoretical understandings already developed by analysing key models which constitute contemporary community work practice. This in turn helps to distinguish community work from other forms of intervention. In this way the chapter acts as a bridge between the theoretical debates of Chapters 5 and 6, and the examination of key themes in community work practice to be presented in Chapter 8.

An extensive review of the community work literature fails to provide an agreed number or the exact scope of different community work models. What has been developed here, therefore, is a discussion that includes the main models and those most readily agreed upon: community care, community organization, community development, community education, community economic development and community action, together with models developed from feminist community work theory, the ethnic minority and anti-racist critique, and the environmentalist and green movement critique which were presented and discussed in Chapter 5. It will be noted that these models have developed, often in an unco-ordinated manner, to address a particular difficulty or concern, or as the application of a particular theory or approach. It needs to be recognized that aspects of these models are not entirely discrete, they are contested and there is a degree of overlap between them. The models are, however, an important method of categorizing central approaches to the activity we call 'community work'. Table 7.1 provides a helpful way of contrasting and comparing the models.

Community care

Community work which is focused on the model of community care attempts to cultivate social networks and voluntary services for, or to be concerned about, the welfare of residents, particularly older people, persons with disabilities, and in many cases children under the age of 5. The community care model, which is also termed 'care in the community', concentrates on developing self-help concepts to address social and welfare needs and uses paid workers (sometimes termed 'organizers') who encourage people to care and to volunteer initiative.

Professional involvement in community care can be on one of three levels. One level is where professionals are expected to fulfil a more or less permanent supportive or monitoring role, using volunteers and low-paid helpers. A second level is where the activity is initiated by professionals who plan to be supportive for only a short period, so that community care can be continued without them. A third level reflects community care as an activity undertaken by laypeople with relatively little help from professionals.

The voluntarism associated with the community care model supports the notion of engaging volunteers in care-giving and advocacy schemes. In reality, there may be concerns over the level of training of volunteers, their reliability and their trustworthiness. Similarly, there may be concern about the exploitation of volunteers as unpaid labour, which may also serve to undermine the jobs of paid workers.

The term 'informal care' refers to care undertaken by families, neighbours and friends, on an informal, unpaid basis and largely in the recipients' own homes. The important contribution of this sector to the British economy and to its social life has been recognized for some time. Just over two million adults received informal care in the UK in 2010, the value of which has been estimated to be £61.7 billion per year or 4.2 per cent of GDP (www.ons.gov. uk/ons/rel/wellbeing/household-satellite-accounts/valuing-informal-adult-care-in-the-uk/art-adult-care.html#tab-abstract, accessed 3 March 2014).

Table 7.1 Models of community work practice

	Strategy	Main role/title of worker	Examples of work/agencies	Selected critical key texts
Community care	Cultivating social networks and voluntary services Developing self-help concepts Campaigning	Organizer, volunteer	Work with older people, persons with disabilities, children under 5 years	Alcock et al. (2008) Trevithick (2012)
Community organization	Improving co-ordination between different welfare agencies	Organizer, catalyst, manager	Councils for Voluntary Service Settlements	Rothman (1970) Alinsky (1971) Beck and Purcell (2013)
Community development	Assisting groups to acquire the skills and confidence to improve quality of life Active participation	Enabler Neighbourhood worker Facilitator	Community groups Tenants groups Settlements	Craig et al. (2011) Gilchrist and Taylor (2011) Ledwith (2011)
Community education	Attempts to bring education and community into a closer and more equal relationship	Educator Facilitator	Community schools/colleges 'Compensatory education' Working-class/feminist adult education	Allen and Martin (1992) Freire (1970; 1972; 1976; 1985) Lovett et al. (1983) Rogers (1994) Tett (2006)
Community action	Usually class-based, conflict-focused, direct action at local level	Activist	Squatting movement Welfare rights movement Resistance against planning and redevelopment Tenants' action	CDP literature (see Appendix) Craig et al. (1982) Jacobs and Popple (1994) Lees and Mayo (1984)

(Continued)

Table 7.1 Continued

Strategy	Main role/title of worker	Examples of work/agencies	Selected critical key texts
Community economic development	Establishing local-based, 'not-for-profit' businesses and cooperatives	Facilitators Development workers	Credit unions	Morris et al. (2013)
Feminist community work	Improvement of women's welfare Working collectively to challenge and eradicate inequalities suffered by women	Activist Enabler Facilitator	Women's refuges Women's health groups Women's therapy centres	Dominelli (2002; 2006) Emejulu (2011) Ledwith (2011)
Ethnic minority and anti-racist community work	Setting up and running groups that support the needs of ethnic minority groups and communities Challenging racism	Activist Volunteer	Autonomous ethnic minority community-based groups	Shukra (2007) Soni (2011)
Environmentalism and the green movement critique	Working with and setting up groups and networks that focus on empowering communities to address climate change, sustainable development and climate justice	Activist Volunteer	Community co-ops	Smith (1998) Dobson and Bell (2006) Reid et al. (2009)

When the first edition of *Analysing Community Work* was published in 1995, the informal care figure was £21.5 billion per year. Such calculations are very difficult to substantiate with any accuracy as the defining feature of this sector is its informal and largely hidden nature. This calculation takes no account of the additional expenditures (travel, adaptions, etc.) or of the opportunity costs in terms of careers and wages forgone by carers. Neither does it take any account of costs of childcare. The figure is useful, however, if only to offer an illustration of this sector's contribution in comparison to total government expenditure on social services which in 2001–12 amounted to £17.2 billion (www.hscic.gov.uk/catalogue/PUB09820/pss-exp-eng-11-12-fin-rpt.pdf, accessed 3 March 2014).

In the last three decades, the encouragement of community care schemes has been given priority by governments as they attempt to rein in public expenditure, and encourage the development of the independent and private sector while trying to develop practical support for carers. The National Health Service and Community Care Act 1990 was to prove an important milestone in the development of community care as it introduced market forces into the provision of health and welfare service provision. This is often referred to as the 'mixed economy of welfare'. Whereas previously social service departments provided and delivered services based on assessed need, legislation now requires them to spend at least 85 per cent of their income on services from the private, voluntary, and independent sector.

Since 1990, and particularly under the Labour government of 1997–2010, there has been a revolution in community care. One was due to the introduction of the 'personalization agenda' and the other was the result of the dismantling of social services departments. (For a detailed discussion of these major changes, see Trevithick 2012.)

Numerous studies have supported the view that women are much more likely to be engaged in community care than men (Dominelli 2002). These findings are also reported by Parker (1981), who states that to talk about community or family care is to 'disguise reality':

> In fact, . . . 'care by the community' almost always means care by family members with little support from others in the 'community'. Further care by family members almost always means care by female members with little support from other relatives. It appears that 'shared care' is uncommon; once one person has been identified as the main carer, other relatives withdraw.
>
> (Parker 1981: 30)

Research data confirms that 58 per cent of carers are women, while the number of people providing more than 50 hours of care every week is 1.3 million (www.carersuk.org, accessed 17 August 2014).

Community care policies have been criticized by a number of social policy writers who point to the dominance of familist ideology, and its links with the wider ideology of possessive individualism (Alcock et al. 2008). They argue that community care has been actively promoted by the political Right in order to avoid the expense of institutional care, but also because this form of care is perceived as the most 'appropriate' and 'natural' form of care for the dependant. This view is derived from the residualist or anti-collectivist approach to welfare whereby the family is seen as the locus of care, and the role of the statutory sector only comes into play when that unit has broken down in some way.

Considerable discussion has been allocated here to the community care model. This is because over the last 30 years and more, the model has developed as a significant and relatively well-resourced form of community work which has clear connections with the ascendancy and influence of the neo-liberal ideology and its drive to reduce state funding of welfare services and to encourage the growth of private care. However, it needs to be noted that since the 1960s a number of social scientists have developed a critique of the failure of institutional care to provide people with humane treatment and have advocated support for individuals in the community (Goffman 1961; Townsend 1962; Foucault 1967; 1977).

Community organization

Community work framed on the community organization model has historically been used widely in Britain as a means of improving the co-ordination between different welfare agencies. Through such co-ordination it is thought possible to avoid duplication of services and lack of resources, while attempting to provide an efficient and effective delivery of welfare. Examples of community organizations are the councils of voluntary service (see, for example, www.bournemouthcvs.org.uk/, accessed 4 March 2014), older persons welfare committees, and 'similar organizations that are engaged in the coordination, promotion and development of the work of a number of bodies in a particular field at local, regional or national levels' (Jones 1977: 6). The community organization model, which tends to be service-orientated, has been engaged in pioneering and experimental work and has often led in more economically less challenged times to the state funding and managing the services developed by such organizations. However, since the banking crisis of 2008–09 and the introduction of government austerity measures, we are aware that though community organizations have been shown to make a significant social and economic contribution to life in the UK, they are finding their funding opportunities are declining (Kane et al. 2014).

In recent years there has been an advance of the campaigning community organization, Citizens UK. Founded in 1989 by Neil Jameson, who was influenced by his training and work with the Industrial Areas Foundation in the USA, Citizens UK was initially known as London Citizens but, according to its website, it is now operating in a number of other cities and hence its change of title (www.citizensuk.org/, accessed 4 March 2014). The organization has brought together a range of groups and individuals and has been involved in campaigns such as that to introduce a living wage (rather than a minimum wage) and has established an Independent Asylum Commission, which is investigating concerns at the way refugees and asylum seekers are treated by the UK Borders Agency.

Critics of the traditional localized community organization model include Dearlove (1974), who presents a class analysis and argues the role of community organizations is to employ 'expert' professionals, whose job it is to offer advice to working-class people in an attempt to stifle the anger and frustration felt in a particular neighbourhood or community. The role of the 'expert' in this model is to channel these feelings into acceptable and approved structures. The Community Development Projects were also critical of the community organization model, arguing, for instance, that the Urban Deprivation Unit created by the Department of the Environment in 1973 was based on the model, and was operating with managerialist methods, and ignoring the needs and concerns of people living in the communities they professed to serve (CDP 1977).

Community organizing is well established in the USA and its theory and practice have been influenced by a number of writers, including Rothman (1970), who identified three distinct types of community organizing: (1) locality development; (2) social action; and (3) social planning. In more recent years there have been studies of community organizing in the USA, including a valuable text by Mondros and Wilson (1994). The view in the USA is that organized community groups can play an important role in influencing government and corporations and they have instituted direct action tactics such as petitions, picketing and boycotting. However, there is also an underlying focus on building organizations which are vehicles for other developments in neighbourhoods and cities. We have also noted the more radical tradition of community organizing with our discussion of the work of Saul Alinsky in Chapter 3 and Chapter 6 and this is further referred to in Chapter 9 with the work of Beck and Purcell (2013).

Community development

The community development model of community work is probably the best known of the approaches and a great deal has been written about it.

Community development is fundamentally a broad approach to working with groups and individuals to help them acquire the skills and confidence to improve the quality of the lives of its members and communities. With its emphasis on promoting self-help by means of education, this model perhaps best reflects the soul of community work.

The community development model, which was championed in North America in the early 1960s by Biddle and Biddle (1965), evolved in the UK from the work initiated by Batten (1957; 1962; 1965; 1967) which, as discussed in Chapter 3, initially derived from his experiences with such a model when working in the British colonies. We also noted that this model of community work was used as a tool by British administrations overseas to harness the local communities into colonial domination. The rationale for the model being used by the British Colonial Office can be seen in HMSO (1954), while a similar notion is given in the UN statement on community development in developing countries (United Nations 1959: 1). The use of the community development model in developing countries has been criticized by a number of commentators, including Ng (1988), who documents how the model was used in the colonies to integrate indigenous people into subordinate positions within the dominant colonizing system.

Community development in Britain has been characterized by intervention at the neighbourhood level and, as noted earlier, has focused upon a process whereby community groups are encouraged to articulate their problems and needs. The expectation is that this will encourage local people to engage in civic collective action in the determination and meeting of these needs. Most but not all community development projects are located in areas of high social and economic need, and practitioners are employed by public bodies, in particular, local authorities, and voluntary and non-governmental organizations (Pitchford 2008; Craig et al. 2011).

As we will see in Chapter 8, the majority of community development workers are women, many of whom have written about their field-work experiences. For example, a black woman, Anionwu (1990), has written about her community development work in relation to a marginalized health problem, sickle cell anaemia. Anionwu believes that the community development approach was successful in enabling her to meet and work with discriminated black sufferers, which led to her setting up the Brent Sickle Cell and Thalassic Centre. Similarly, Ledwith (2011) provides a number of examples of women engaged in community development while Gilchrist (1992) presents a commentary on her experiences as a community worker in an inner-city area of Bristol.

Community development has built an international profile through the International Association for Community Development, whose administrative offices are presently located in the UK; also through the US-based Community Development Society; and through the *Community Development Journal*, all of which are discussed in Chapter 9, which will also present a case study of a community development project in Hong Kong.

Gilchrist and Taylor (2011) have identified three central features of community development: (1) informal education; (2) collective action; and (3) organization development. With regard to informal education, they maintain that people learn new skills 'through taking on tasks, observing others, "having a go" and receiving feedback' (2011: 10). According to Gilchrist and Taylor, the collective action aspect of community development comes about through people identifying the aims they have in common and then provides 'the impetus to mobilise community members to develop a joint plan of action, recruit allies and activists and decide what needs to be done to make the changes they want' (2011: 11).

Finally, the organization development aspect of community development 'means helping it to evolve a form that enables the members to achieve their goals, to act legally and to be accountable to the membership and wider community' (2011: 11).

Two key themes of community development are group process and achieving set goals. A group cannot successfully accomplish one of these key themes without accomplishing the other. The role of the community development worker is to help facilitate this progression in order that the group can attain its stated objectives. This facilitation can move from indirect approaches or a 'non-directive' style of work to a more direct intervention or leadership role. The skill of the worker is to decide when and how best to deploy the right approach, which needs constant reflection. We will be looking in more detail at skills in Chapter 8 when we examine practice.

Ledwith's approach to community development is a radical one. In her paper 'Reclaiming the radical agenda: a critical approach to community development', Ledwith argues that the activity needs to be informed by the unity of theory and practice and where there is a synthesis between the two (see www.infed.org/community/critical_community_development.htm, accessed 17 March 2014). Ledwith maintains that community development should be inspired by a vision of social and environmental justice and where local practice is situated 'within the wider political picture'. This is a valuable contribution to our thinking on community development which further strengthens the argument made in previous chapters to develop an activity that resonates with the challenges now being faced by communities in the twenty-first century. (See also Emejulu and Shaw 2010.)

An analysis of community development in Ireland is made by Powell and Geoghegan (2004), who argue that it had become a vehicle for assisting local regeneration. Arguing that the political Right has a powerful grip on Irish society, the authors suggest that, despite this:

> Partnership may be the only democratic means of influencing long-term social change in Ireland that is genuinely inclusive. The goal of

community development is to 'democratise democracy' in a genuinely socially inclusive form. In a globalised society, dominated by the market, that is a task of Herculean proportions. Yet there is ample evidence of citizens willing to try. That must be the hope of our civilization.

(Powell and Geoghegan, 2004: 272)

Finally, it is possible to access and view a range of videos that reflect the breadth and diversity of community development in the UK and internationally at www.mashpedia.com/Community_development, accessed 17 March 2014.

Community education

The community education model of community work has been described as 'a significant attempt to redirect educational policy and practice in ways which bring education and community into a closer and more equal relationship' (Allen et al. 1987: 2). Community education has a long tradition in the United Kingdom which, according to Martin (1987), has developed from three main strands. The first is the school-based village and community college movement, initiated by Henry Morris in Cambridgeshire during the late 1920s (Morris 1925). (For a discussion of the life and work of Morris, see Ree 1973; 1985; McCloy 2013.) This was followed by the establishment of similar integrated educational provision in Leicestershire under the guidance of Stewart Mason in the following decade (Fairbairn 1979). The second strand of community education was the experiments developing from the Educational Priority Area projects (1969–72) which attempted to provide 'compensatory education' in selected disadvantaged inner-city areas as recommended by the DES (1967). (For a detailed discussion of these experiments, see Halsey 1972; Midwinter 1972; 1975.) The third strand was the working-class adult education work undertaken by a number of the Community Development Projects in the late 1960s and the early 1970s (for examples, see Lovett 1975; Lovett et al. 1983).

Community education has been further analysed as having three 'qualitatively different ideologies': consensus, pluralism, and conflict (Martin 1987: 22). Martin argues that the consensus or universal model is focused on the secondary school/community college; the pluralist or reformist model is linked to primary schools and their neighbourhoods; and the conflict or radical model is focused on working-class action. To the three ideologies outlined above we can be add the feminist analysis of community education which is presented by Rogers (1994).

The conflict or radical model shares with community development an emphasis on innovative, informal, political education, and has been greatly influenced by the Brazilian adult educator, Paulo Freire, whose work has served as a significant challenge to school-based education. We discussed Freire's contribution to community work theory in Chapter 6, which includes his key argument that the dominant approach to education is based on the 'banking' system which considers knowledge to be a commodity that needs to be accumulated in order to gain access to positions of authority and power. As we noted, Freire articulated a view that education can be constructed for liberation where learners and teachers engage in a process in which abstract and concrete knowledge, together with experience, are integrated into *praxis* (which can be defined as action intended to alter the material and social world). The fundamental features of this praxis are critical thinking and dialogue (as opposed to discussion), which seek to challenge conventional explanations of everyday life, while at the same time considering the action necessary for the transformation of oppressive conditions.

In more recent years community education in the UK has been expanded to take in the notion of lifelong learning and development and social inclusion. This is principally so in Scotland, examples of which are presented in the work by McConnell (2002). Further, Tett (2006), who also writes about developments in Scotland, explains that community education is a concept with a political role, purpose and practice. In her examination of a number of community education projects, Tett argues that there is a need to look beyond the policy speech-making to recognize and explore some of the tensions in policy developments. Tett is critical of the view that social marginalization is an individual problem but instead maintains it is the result of structured inequalities. Her view is that community education and lifelong learning should have as one of its key focuses democratic renewal.

Community action

In our consideration in previous chapters, we established that the community action model of community work was both a reaction to the more paternalistic forms of community work and a response by relatively powerless groups to increase their effectiveness. We have also discussed the way in which the Community Development Projects were initiated as a government-supported community work venture in the 1960s and 1970s based upon the community organization and community development models. Soon after their commencement, this direction changed, with the projects evolving on the lines of the community action model.

The community action model (which has also been termed the social action model) of community work has traditionally been class-based and uses conflict and direct action, usually at a local level, in order to negotiate with power holders over what is often a single issue. Early writings on community action by, among others, Lapping (1970), Leonard (1975), Radford (1970) and Silburn

(1971), together with the influential community work series of books published by Routledge & Kegan Paul in conjunction with the Association of Community Workers (Mayo and Jones 1974; Jones and Mayo 1975; Mayo 1977; Curno 1978; Craig et al. 1979; 1982; Smith and Jones 1981; Ohri et al. 1982), as well as a number of other significant writings (for example, Cockburn 1977; Cowley et al. 1977; O'Malley 1977; Curno et al. 1982; Lees and Mayo 1984) provide a rich source of examples of the practice and debates surrounding the model during the late 1960s, 1970s and early 1980s. The North American community work literature also contains examples and discussions of community or social action. The texts that have been the most influential in the United Kingdom include Alinsky (1969; 1971); Lamoureux et al. (1989) and Piven and Cloward (1977).

Since the 1960s, examples of community action have been varied and include the squatting movement, the welfare rights movement (including the Claimants Union), and different forms of resistance against planning and redevelopment. Mayo (1982) believes the most typical form of community action in the 1960s and 1970s in the UK was focused around the issue of repairs and maintenance of council housing. This view is reflected in the literature. For instance, in the early 1980s, the now defunct Association of Community Workers devoted a publication to community work and tenant action (Henderson et al. 1982), and considerable space was allocated to housing-related issues in the now obsolete magazine, *Community Action.*

During the 1970s an important strand of community action was linked with trade union activity (see, for example, Corkey and Craig 1978; Craig et al. 1979). This was often as a direct result of the work of the Community Development Projects in a particular locality. Examples of the projects that arose from such an intervention include the Coventry Workshop, the Tyneside Trade Union Studies Unit, and the Joint Docklands Action Group. This type of action was further developed in the 1980s and 1990s by municipal socialism, which was based on a broad political group described as the 'new urban left'. Towards the end of the existence of the Greater London Council (GLC) (which was dissolved by the Thatcher government in 1986), there were a plethora of GLC-supported community projects. At the time, however, Goodwin and Duncan (1986) argued that such policies are most effective in terms of polit- ical mobilization and that policy-makers on the Left had to be aware of the constraints and limitations of policies promising large-scale job creation and local economic regeneration. With rising unemployment, the issue of community action and the problems faced by people without employment became an increasing concern during the early 1980s and continued through the 1990s (Ohri and Roberts 1981; Purcell 1982; Gallacher et al. 1983; Cumella 1984; Salmon 1984; McMichael et al. 1990), while community action and housing co-operatives have also been an important theme (*Roof* 1986).

Since the 1990s the term community action has been co-opted by a range of groups, many of which have little or nothing to do with challenging and negotiating with power brokers and are often focused on local small-scale 'safe' activities such as volunteering and training (see, for example, www. communityactionderby.org.uk/, accessed 17 March 2014). At the same time a UK party political organization, the Community Action Party, based in Warrington, Lancashire, has emerged to put up candidates at local council elections. This co-option of the term community action is not unusual and reflects its lack of precision for many in local communities.

The role of the community worker in the more radical community action model is an interesting one and highlights the tension in government towards community work. We have noted in previous discussions that the majority of community work is sponsored by the state which, through its agencies, will define, supervise and regulate the work of practitioners. However, community action, by its very nature, is often engaged in conflict with the employers of community workers, i.e., the local authorities. A wider debate on the contradictions surrounding this position is addressed in *In and Against the State* (London Edinburgh Weekend Return Group 1980). It is for this reason that community action is usually seen as an area of practice undertaken by campaigners and activists who are not employed, directly or indirectly, by the state. Thomas (1983) argues that one cannot combine the role of community worker with that of community activist. They are, in his view, different, and clearly reflect his own adherence to the pluralist approach and practice theories:

> Community work interventions require a certain degree of experience and training; they offer specific skills and knowledge to a community or agency which are different from (though not inherently better than and often over lapping with) those offered by local residents who take on active roles within community groups.
>
> (Thomas 1983: 11)

In the same book, which reviews the evolution of community work, Thomas does not consider the role of community action other than in passing reference. Instead he focuses on community work as a specialist occupation, with 'a particular and limited intervention' (Thomas 1983: 7), located in neighbourhoods and agencies. The decision by Thomas not to address the community action model highlights his view that community work is a profession, rather than a political activity.

Community economic development

In the past 20 years there has been increasing recognition that the UK economy is one of the most centralized in Europe. In response, there has been growing attention paid to how this can be addressed through community economic development (CED), which is focused on strengthening local economies and local groups. This approach is well developed in the USA and Canada. For example, the Western Economic Diversification Canada (WD) has made a significant contribution to CED in Canadian urban centres and rural areas by encouraging regional approaches to economic development through partnerships with non-profit-making organizations and community groups. The organization has also designed and delivered community development programmes to help build community capacity, enhance knowledge and skills, and renew and sustain rural and urban communities. In the past few years WD has invested millions of dollars of federal funds to support CED and to deliver services and programmes that are efficient and accountable and, importantly, can maximize the benefits for individual communities (see www.wd.gc.ca/eng/106.asp, accessed 26 March 2014).

While CED is not as developed in the UK, there is evidence that the growth in inequality is linked with economic centralization (Wilkinson and Pickett 2010; Lansley 2011). In particular, material produced by Jenkins (2004) demonstrates that the centralization of economic power in the UK, with increasing corporate dominance and centralized decision-making, is damaging local initiatives. On the positive side there are organizations such as the Institute for New Economic Thinking, the Business Alliance for Local Living Economies, and the New Economics Foundation, which are challenging economic orthodoxy and arguing for a fundamental move away from the status quo to approaches that are more inclusive and localized. One of these approaches is CED, which in the UK has been defined as 'economic development led by people within the community and based on local knowledge and local action, with the aim of creating economic opportunities and better social conditions locally' (Morris et al. 2013: 5).

According to Morris et al. (2013), there is currently evidence that CED can generate higher levels of local job creation, particularly in disadvantaged areas as well as increase local governance, which promotes civic engagement. However, they also argue there remains much to be done to persuade local authorities and political leaders of the benefits of CED as well as the need to encourage banks to remove their discrimination towards lending to small locally owned businesses and co-operatives.

One area of work where CED can play a part is in the creation and support of credit unions, which can provide credit or loans at competitive rates, offering a good return on savings as well as financial services to their members. Credit unions are community-based 'not-for-profit' organizations that are intended to serve their members rather than make profits as conventional banks are driven to do. This means credit unions are able to reach out to those usually excluded from financial services, which in turn can assist in boosting economic activity at a local level. Credit unions working alongside community development projects have been successful in many countries, as they can support sustainable development and increase local economic activity.

Community work and in particular community development have often focused on the social aspects of building networks and networking, encouraging social capital and building more resilient communities through increasing skills and knowledge. The approaches within CED which can include community economic enterprises, development trusts, co-operatives and social enterprises offers a further way of achieving these goals while addressing the need to challenge the monopolistic power of corporations and in their place develop localized groups that are based on establishing a more just and sustainable economy.

Feminist community work

Chapters 4 and 6 outlined the evolution of feminist community work theory based on the development, since the 1960s, of feminist theory. Female community workers have applied these theoretical understandings to practice (see, for example, Dixon et al. 1982), both in feminist campaigns and in permeating existing community work practice and principles (Dominelli 2002; 2006; Ledwith 2011). While there is no agreed single theoretical feminist position, there is a consensus that the central aim of feminist community work practice is the improvement of women's welfare by collectively challenging the social determinants of women's inequality. Although much of the practice is focused at the personal, local or neighbourhood level, it is linked practically and theoretically with wider feminist concerns. For example, women have been active in many localities in providing accommodation, usually in the form of emergency housing, for women suffering from domestic abuse. This securement of safe accommodation is a response to the immediate suffering experienced by individual women at the hands of violent men, to the inadequate provision made by the state for such women, as well as presenting a stand against male violence.

Chapter 6 discussed the central role of the women's movement as a feature of new social movements, and how feminist campaigns are an example of practice that links local work with that undertaken at national level. As well as the example of local women's refuges, which are affiliated to the national Women's Aid organization, we can note a number of other campaigns and networks which have both a local and a national profile. These include women's health groups; women's involvement in the 1984–85 miners strike; and campaigns to improve and increase childcare facilities.

As well as the commitment to working collectively to challenge and eradicate inequalities suffered by women, feminist community work practice emphasizes the objective of working with women's own personal experiences in groups. This approach avoids the individualizing and pathologizing methods often used by social workers and therapists to interpret the issues presented by women.

This work is often undertaken in the form of consciousness-raising groups which were mentioned in our earlier discussion of feminist community work theory. Women's consciousness-raising groups are intended to break down feelings of isolation and provide participants with a sense of solidarity in order to engage in co-operative struggles. As we have seen above, consciousness-raising groups can also be used to provide women with the strength, knowledge and skills to challenge professionals' definition of their positions. Overall, these groups are considered by feminist community workers as an important first step in the process of change; it is a necessary but not sufficient condition for the transformation of social relations.

The use of women-only groups, whether in specialist consciousness-raising or in more general ways, is a central feature of feminist community work. Among its advocates, Hanmer and Statham (1988) argue that the quality of the group process is likely to be improved in a single-sex group, because the intimate and interpersonal problems are likely to be confronted more quickly. The authors claim that the realization that their problems are not unique should help to reduce women's feelings of personal inadequacy, and thus start to alleviate isolation and stigmatization. Similarly, research has shown that men take over and influence community groups by controlling the 'introduction and pursuit of topics, the use of available time, the lack of emotional content in conversation' (Hanmer and Statham 1988: 131).

Feminist community workers have engaged in a variety of creative attempts to develop non-hierarchical structures and more participatory ways of working. Criticisms of traditional forms of organization as being alienating and inaccessible initially resulted in attempts to develop structureless groups. However, there is recognition that it is 'a mistake to equate structure with hierarchy' (Freeman 1984: 62). This has led one writer to argue that 'the quest for a structure which is genuinely participatory, which does not alienate people, and yet achieves the goals which the group has set itself must be central to feminist practice within the women's movement and in community work' (Barker 1986: 87).

Similarly, process models in group work have been of concern to feminist community workers who indicate that they can function to exclude and to intimidate group members. Process models are concerned with both the different stages a group moves through (for instance, reflection, planning and action) and the development individual group members achieve. According to Brown (1992), process models have two ideologically different positions. One emphasizes individual emotional growth and development. The other model is founded upon political and social philosophies and is engaged in achieving change for disadvantaged people. Previously the importance of process has been overlooked by radical community work because of the dominance of the former model. Dixon et al. (1982) argue, for instance, that this non-political approach was reflected in the writings of early theorists, such as Batten. However, as they go on to state, 'Feminist analysis shows clearly that process is political, and needs urgent consideration if our campaigns are to achieve their aims' (1982: 63).

In 2011, the *Community Development Journal* published a special issue focusing on feminisms and contemporary community development. One of the articles in this special issue by Emejulu (2011) provides a valuable analysis and critique of the way in which writers have positioned feminist community development around elements of 'community', 'power' and 'equality', which has, according to the author, ignored (unintentionally) opportunities to deploy feminist political theory to understand 'women' as political actors. Emejulu (2011) then uses a post-structuralist discourse analysis to re-theorize the core constitutive elements of feminist community development in the UK. The author's intention is to help rethink our understanding of feminist community development so that it can 'more effectively position itself in the broader politics of radical democratic pluralism and the on-going fight for respect, recognition and social justice for groups at the margins' (Emejulu 2011).

Ethnic minority and anti-racist community work

Chapter 5 discussed how traditional forms of community work have failed both to meet the particular needs of the ethnic minority communities in the UK and to effectively challenge institutional and personal racism. It also discussed the response to this by the ethnic minority communities and those community workers who are engaged in developing an anti-racist critique.

Historically there is substantial evidence that ethnic minority communities in the UK have not passively accepted racism and racist policy and practice. Since their arrival in Britain, people from ethnic minorities have been active in their communities, supporting each other and organizing to resist discrimination and defend their rights (Bhavnani et al. 2005). The focus of discrimination has varied, nevertheless ethnic minorities have been and continue to be disadvantaged in a number of sectors, including certain areas of education, housing, health, employment, police relations and immigration. Similarly, a range of different and overlapping responses has developed from ethnic minority communities, including campaigns; self-help groups; direct action; and alternative and supplementary provision. At times these have required coalitions to be built and alliances forged, at others autonomous organization has been preferred.

There is also evidence of people from minority groups having historically been excluded from mainstream political life in Britain, though at the time of writing there are 27 serving ethnic minority MPs in the House of Commons which is 4.2 per cent of the total of those sitting in the 'lower house'. As we have noted elsewhere, the UK population is becoming increasingly diverse in terms of ethnicity. Nevertheless though the numbers of ethnic minority MPs increased by 15 between the 2001 and 2010 General Elections, with the Labour Party having more representatives from ethnic minorities than other parties, the diversity of MPs is still disproportionate to the general population. If the House of Commons were to truly represent proportionately the numbers of the non-white UK population, there would be around 117 ethnic minority MPs (Wood and Cracknell 2013).

The studies that have been made of the influence of ethnic minority community-based organizations and groups provide useful insights. For instance, the work by Gouldbourne (1998) indicates that certain autonomous black community-based groups have over time successfully influenced mainstream institutions by placing on the political agenda contentious issues, such as police relations with ethnic minority communities and the education of ethnic minority children. Cheetham (1988) meanwhile argues that ethnic minority associations in Britain have a vitality and energy that have assisted their development as active self-help groups. Kalka (1991) discusses the tension between entrenched local organizations and newly founded ethnic associations and pressure groups. The author describes the situation in the London Borough of Harrow where Gujarati Hindus became increasingly articulate in presenting demands and acquiring new skills to assert their position.

Other research that describes and discusses the role of, and work with, ethnic minority community-based groups includes that by Sondhi (1982). Writing about his work at the Asian Resource Centre in the multi-racial community of Handsworth in Birmingham, Sondhi views the agency as a campaigning one that provides a much needed advice and information service in the locality. The agency also undertook specific work with the Asian elderly (Asian Sheltered Residential Accommodation 1981).

The establishment of community projects by the ethnic minority population is often a response to exclusion from white-dominated provision as well as providing opportunities to develop and strengthen cultural, social and political ties. Although people from ethnic minorities do not form a homogeneous group in Britain, they share with each other the experience of racism and of colonization which, as we noted earlier, has given them certain strengths and perspectives.

Perhaps the major policy change that has impacted most directly on Muslims, and indirectly on other minority groups living in the UK, has been the government policies introduced in the aftermath of the 9/11 attacks in the USA on 11 September 2001. This was followed by the 7/7 bombings in London on 7 July 2005 and has led to increased anti-terrorist legislation and law enforcement powers. It was soon after these events that UK social policy, that had been based on the concept of 'race relations', moved to one focused on the notion of community cohesion (Worley 2005), which has primarily been concerned with the state increasing internal security. This has included advocating that people from ethnic minorities should adopt the ill-defined and politically contentious sense of 'Britishness'. If this means democracy, fairness, justice, freedom of speech and personal security, then research has indicated these values are equally shared by new migrants, resident minorities and the majority population (Rutter et al. 2007). The move to policies of community cohesion is a further development of the attempts in the 1960s to 1970s to assimilate minorities into the British way of life, which was followed by different approaches to multiculturalism. Some are concerned, however, that the contemporary debates on community cohesion is 'winding the clock' back to the ill-fated assimilation policies of this period (Flynn and Craig 2012) which failed to recognize that multicultural societies are a way of life (Parekh 2000). According to Shukra (2007: 7):

> The language and framework of community cohesion are a managerial one that seeks to contain and direct people's lives by reducing difference. It is at the expense of people's freedom to forge their own identities, relationships and solidarities in the process of challenging oppression and discrimination.

Finally, there is growing concern globally that the conflicts in the Middle East are increasing the phenomenon of Islamophobia. The research by Sheridan (2006) reports a significant increase in the negative experiences felt by Muslims in the UK since the events of 9/11. Further, Mukhopadhyay (2007: 102) points to the emergence of alarmist media reports that 'depicts a Europe flooded by Muslims in the form of legal and illegal immigrants'. The evidence is, however, that British Muslim youth are now one of the most deprived and alienated in the community and the British Muslim population generally experiences the highest rate of unemployment, has the highest rate of ill-health, and experiences the highest proportion of those without qualifications (Roberts 2006). The effect of this is well described by Soni (2011) who states that:

> In such circumstances that clearly include unacceptable levels of deprivation, hostility from those outside the community, a lack of real cohesion within the Muslim community (in spite of perceptions which perhaps suggest the converse) and the possible attraction of ready-made 'masculine' identities which particularly provide a convenient means of uniting some young Muslims under the guise of protecting their religion, it is not surprising that notions of religious pride and honour are triggered.
>
> (2011: 65)

Environmentalism and the green movement critique

We discussed in Chapter 5 the emergence and strengthening of the environmentalism and green movement critique which has become the focus of a number of community work projects both in the UK and globally. Environmentalism and the green movement form a broad ideology and practice and it would be difficult here to provide more than a brief comment on them as a model for community work.

Environmental issues such as air and water pollution, carbon emissions, disposing of packaging, resource depletion, energy security, food shortages and GM crops, and the consequences of global warming and climate change impact on us all every day wherever we live. Importantly people are now making a link between these issues and the way we order our economic and political affairs so much so that the central motivating idea for environmental campaigners is that of 'sustainability'. The Millennium Development Goals (MDG), which were agreed by 191 nation states at the United Nations Millennium Summit in 2002, have sustainable development as one of their eight goals.

A feature of the broad environmental and green movement ideology and practice is what Smith (1998) terms ecological citizenship and Dobson and Bell (2006) call environmental citizenship. These ideologies are particularly valuable for community work as they emphasize civil citizenship, political citizenship and social citizenship, all of which resonate with community work's focus on social justice and equality (Cannan 2000). Environmental citizenship goes further and captures the idea of an obligation to future generations to create a sustainable environment and communities. In particular, the model is future-orientated and shuns the short-term nature of neo-liberalism (Smith and Pangsapa 2008). Reid et al. (2009) present a vision of how best we can develop practices that do not damage the environment in our daily life. Using a sequential mixed methods approach to research which included participants keeping a daily diary, the authors show how reflexivity can help change behaviour and develop ways of living that do not compromise the environment in our local communities.

Conclusion

In conclusion, we can see that although there is overlap between the models discussed, particularly in terms of the techniques and skills used, the models reflect the different traditions, ideologies and emerging ideas and movements that we have been considering in previous chapters. Community care, community organization and community economic development represent the pluralist tradition in community work. The community action model and the models from feminism, ethnic minority and anti-racist critique, and the environmentalism and green movement critique reflect aspects of the radical and socialist approach which emerged in the 1960s. Different aspects of community development and community education fit into these diverse approaches. For example, in the case of community education, the radical strand of the model is epitomized in the work of Freire and of Lovett. The work of school-based community education, including the compensatory education programmes, is, however, an example of the pluralist approach. Certain models, for instance, community care, are centred upon the premise of delivering a service in a more efficient and often cost-effective or cost-saving manner. Other models, such as those that reflect the radical and social-ist approaches, are focused around certain ideological positions and commit-ments. Together with the remaining models, the above offers us a framework with which to understand community work practice.

One important question that emerges from the discussion on the theories of community work and the above discussion on models is whether all those employed as community workers in organizations practising the pluralist models are in total agreement with the aspirations offered by such models. For instance, socialist feminists, who have a particular view of society and on how it should be organized, may be employed in community care, pluralist community education, and other community work positions. Traditionally, workers in these areas are required to act in a 'neutral' manner and to develop formal links with policy-makers in order to improve services for a particular community in a manner which endorses the status quo. This tension which was so well presented in the seminal work *In and Against the State* (London Edinburgh Weekend Return Group 1980) remains an enduring one for the community work community.

Questions

---

1 What community work models resonate best with your understanding of the activity? Explain why.
2 Are there further models of community work which could be added to those presented here?

---

8 Community work in practice

Introduction

In Chapter 7 we considered in detail the range of different community work models that reflect the nature and breadth of the activity. We noted that these models provide us with an important method of relating the theoretical discussions generated in Chapters 5 and 6 to various forms of community work practice. Together these three chapters have provided us with a detailed account and a clearer understanding of the significant constituent elements of community work theory and practice.

The aim of this chapter is to link this developing discussion with a number of central practice themes that have been generated at various stages in this book but which we have not been able to discuss in detail: community work values; skills; education and training; the employment of community workers; and management. We begin by reflecting on the value base of community work.

Community work values

Throughout this book we have been alerted to the central values of community work, which include the need to work in a collective manner in order to address economic and social injustice, inequality and to advance the theory and practice of anti-discrimination. These values have emerged and established themselves in the community work field over time and have been agreed upon by practitioners and activists, and those whose main role has been to teach, research and to write about the activity. For example, the UK National Occupational Standards for Community Development (FCDL 2009) states that there are five key values:

- Equality and Anti-discrimination
- Social Justice

- Collective Action
- Community Empowerment
- Working and Learning Together.

It is claimed that a community development practitioner needs to relate these values to their roles and actions in order to effectively address the central issue of the imbalance of power in society.

A central question in our discussion on community work values is, how do our values emerge? In essence, our values have emerged from two powerful forces. One is shaped by the various cultural, moral, religious and political systems and understandings which impact on our daily lives and in which most of us have been brought up. These values are embedded in us and in our society and can be sanctioned through our laws and the legal system. Values also shape and inform the way professions conduct themselves. Ultimately values have a major influence on our individual behaviour, attitudes and the way we deal with particular situations.

In the UK, Christian values and modern secular western liberalism have led to the establishment of particular principles which are considered para-mount for the way our society operates. These include the protection of certain liberties, and the freedom of people to enjoy their own beliefs and activities as long as they do not restrict the freedom of others. Values can be specific to different countries or regions but with the globalizing of economic and social relations, we are arguably witnessing both a coalescing of value systems and a conflict between different value systems.

The other way our personal values emerge is through our own individual experiences which shape our understanding of the world and the part we play in it. This may come about through reflection, from reading and discussion; from participation in community and national life; from life-enhancing experi-ences such as travelling internationally; and from viewing or listening to the media. Our values determine our behaviour in areas such as our personal and sexual relations and our moral position on a number of key questions or issues in contemporary life. Our values can also be shaped by circumstances such as our gender, ethnicity, age, sexuality, our class location and factors relating to disabilities.

Our personal and political values then are a reflection of the way we each view and act in society and by the ideology which informs our daily life. Our values determine how we vote or do not vote, how we argue our position on a range of issues and how we live our daily lives.

As we have seen, community work is a value-driven activity and it is there-fore important to be clear what our values are and how we practise these in the work we undertake. Further, it is vital for these values to be made explicit when engaging in community work, in whatever capacity, as they feed through to our objectives and our practice.

As we noted above, the UK National Occupational Standards for Community Development states that one of the five key values is community action. In the majority of societies, democracy is considered to be the fundamental cornerstone of its citizens' lives and for the most part people feel the need for their views to be heard and for them to be represented in decision-making forums, such as local councils and parliament. However, most countries have what is termed representative democracy which means that individual citizens can only influence political decision-making at a distance. An individual's role is therefore limited to electing political representatives who will make decisions on their behalf. It is against this background that we have seen the emergence of community politics and community action, where people take a more direct route to highlighting their concerns and demanding change. So while it can be argued that democracy is a valuable feature of our societies, it also needs to be recognized it has certain limitations and there are other more localized or relevant forums and forms of action that people can engage in. Therefore, community work with its focus on equality, anti-discrimination and social justice, needs to engage in democracy while recognizing it is a far from perfect way of operating, and hence the need to have at the forefront the key value of community action.

Before moving on to consider the skills needed for community work, it is useful here to refer to the notion of civil society. While recognizing the limitations of democracy we also need to be aware of the potential of civil society, which was highlighted by the work of Antonio Gramsci. As we noted in Chapter 6, Gramsci argued that the state encourages consent in order to sustain the dominant hegemony, but can, when necessary, exercise coercion. Gramsci saw the value of civil society as a set of institutions which has the contradictory role of securing consent while being a vehicle for key forums to challenge the dominant hegemony. So civil society is fundamental to sustaining democracy as it offers a place where opinions can be developed and presented, and for community work it enables the opportunities for the exchange of information, discussion and action.

The role of community development in sustaining and strengthening civil society in Europe is considered by Henderson and Vercseg (2010). The authors reflect on the collapse of communist regimes in a number of Eastern European countries, the impact of the 2008–09 financial recession on different communities, and in the UK the widespread disillusionment with politicians due to the MPs' expenses scandal. The wide-ranging remit the authors give themselves enables them to explore the contribution that community development can make in enhancing the crucial 'space' between the state and the public, in which community groups, social movements and campaigning organizations can exist and thrive.

Community work skills

One of the main features of community work is that it is an 'open occupation', which, according to Smith (1980), gives it a degree of richness, vitality and variety. Likewise, Thomas (1983: 185) argues for the necessity of an 'open occupation' philosophy and policy in order to encourage people from a range of backgrounds to take up community work.

The diversity of backgrounds of those undertaking community work means people bring to the activity an array of skills and knowledge which in turn gives community work its unique and creative position in contemporary life. Before considering the skills that a practitioner might need to success-fully undertake their role, let's look at what we mean by skills.

Generally, skills are divided into two main categories. The first is broad-based skills which we all need to develop in order to sustain our lives and to successfully interact in the world. These include what are often termed life and social skills, such as the ability to successfully manage our time, to respectfully relate to others, and the ability to operate within certain social rules. Other skills are specific to the work we undertake, and for those engaged in community work, they can include skills such as the ability to critically understand the world around us, to understand ourselves and others, to develop trusting and respectful relationships with a wide range of people, and the ability to communicate successfully.

Skills can be learnt, developed and refined and sometimes they can be practised without conscious thought. However, it is crucial that skills are regularly up-dated and enhanced through training and education and through self-reflection and the receipt of accurate supportive feedback from others.

As mentioned already, a detailed and comprehensive text on community work skills is that by Henderson and Thomas (2013), which, with its focus on neighbourhood work and its easily accessible style, is intended for a wider audience than community workers. For example, regeneration officers, youth workers, housing officers, health visitors and health promotion staff are the potential readers of this book.

Henderson and Thomas (2013) identify nine stages that neighbourhood work moves through and allocate a section in the book to each. These stages are: (1) entering the neighbourhood; (2) getting to know the neighbourhood, what next?; (3) needs, goals and roles; (4) making contacts and bringing people together; (5) forming and building organizations; (6) helping to clarify goals and priorities; (7) keeping the organization going; (8) dealing with friends and enemies; and (9) leavings and endings. These different stages suggest different skills required by the worker, for example, making contacts, including meeting members of a community in order to identify their interest in collective action and the contribution and role they might make; group work; locality development; negotiation, particularly with decision-makers; and a combination of an understanding of political processes and practical political skills.

Another useful and comprehensive skills manual is that produced by Harris (2009). This edition is an up-dated version of one also edited by Harris in 1994 and published by the now defunct Association of Community Workers. The new edition is written *by* community workers and activists *for* community workers and activists, and differs from previous versions because it contains case studies presenting green themes and environmental issues while still covering tried and tested ideas across all aspects of community work. It covers a number of topics including:

- Identifying community needs – undertaking research
- Making contact with communities of interest and identity
- Helping groups decide what resources they need
- How to get resources
- Funding and fundraising
- Creating alliances
- Building effective relationships – working with other professionals
- Supporting community representatives
- Communications within communities and between groups
- Setting up new groups – visioning and developing structures and systems
- Supporting existing groups – planning and taking actions
- Supporting existing groups – managing differences/conflict/group dynamics
- Working with children
- Community work with young people
- Faith-based community work
- ICT for community groups.

To identify and discuss in detail the exact number of skills necessary to effectively undertake community work is beyond the scope of this book and I would refer readers to the texts mentioned above. However, it is possible to identify seven core skills that a community worker will need in their 'skills tool box'. These are not in any particular order, as they need to be viewed as operating in a holistic manner. The skills are:

- A critical understanding of the world around us
- The professional use of self
- Communication skills
- Group work skills

- Planning and organizing skills
- Team working
- Research skills.

Let us consider these in a little more depth.

A critical understanding of the world around us

Before we can effectively assess and intervene in communities, we need to have a critical understanding of the changing economic, political and social structures that impact upon us at the local, national and international levels. Without a critical understanding of the interplay of these key features, we cannot work effectively. For example, we need to be aware of the power imbalances in society; the resultant low income thresholds and widespread poverty in our society; the impact of social exclusion due to a range of inequalities such as health and education; the effect of disadvantage and discrimination; and the creation and labelling of 'social problems'.

To enable us to develop this critical understanding, we need to read critically and widely, to think critically and to engage in activities such as attending relevant conferences, workshops and meetings which encourage critical debate. The key here is to engage in processes and forums which take the debate forward in a manner which is reflective and is understanding of the communities in which we work and live.

The professional use of self

This is a term that has emerged from social work where a number of writers argue that to be an effective practitioner you need to be in touch with your own feelings, have a clear appreciation of one's own values, and an understanding of how we behave and appear to others. It demands staying focused on the present, being aware of our feelings and thoughts while attempting to understand the position of others.

Trevithick (2012) makes the case well when she says that it is the ability to become involved with but not merged with people in the communities we are engaged with:

> It is about allowing ourselves to be affected by the experiences and hardships that people face in ways that move us. In the case of injustice, it can encourage an appropriate *healthy sense of outrage*, which can propel us in our efforts to help bring about change. In emotionally fraught situations, our self-awareness can guide us to take up an appropriate position of separateness, whilst also

maintaining a clear connection . . ., so that we are not too distant or inflexible on the one hand, nor too merged or inappropriately accommodating on the other.

(Trevithick 2012: 111)

In the use of self it is imperative that the practitioner tries to develop and maintain trusting and respectful relationships and in doing so it invites others to do the same.

Communication skills

The skills of being able to listen carefully and respectfully without interrupting others, to write clearly and accurately, and to speak effectively and succinctly are important at all levels of community work. Poor communication can produce misunderstandings and a community worker therefore needs to keep focused on the most appropriate means of communication in order to find mutual understanding and to ensure the objectives being set can be met. For example, it is important to avoid jargon while communicating clearly and carefully considering the context in which we are speaking or writing.

We need also to appreciate and be sensitive to languages other than English and, where possible, arrange for that to be catered for in communications. Similarly the needs of those with a hearing or sight loss should be respected and addressed and their communication needs accommodated.

Group work skills

The ability to work effectively in different types of groups is a central skill for community work, as so much activity takes place in such forums. Group work has many different meanings and styles, particularly in the therapy field, but one of the models that best reflects its use in community work is social group work which focuses on group experiences, to assist its members to manage more successfully challenges in their community. The community worker in this setting is often a facilitator to ensure the group is effective in its focus and allows group members to feel comfortable in a group setting. The focus in such groups is usually to enable individuals to develop the skills both individually and collectively to address their own concerns and also of those in their community. One of the books that has influenced group work thinking and practice in the community work field is that by Brown (1992), while a helpful piece on group work is offered by infed.org, based at George Williams College (http://infed.org/mobi/what-is-groupwork/, accessed 7 April 2014).

Planning and organizing skills

A good deal of a community worker's time is spent engaged in working with community members to set goals, make decisions and plan for action. These tasks all require skills that involve setting objectives, designing a plan to achieve an agreed objective, scheduling resources, managing and organizing time and deciding upon priorities. The decision-making involves gathering relevant information, evaluating its use and choosing between opportunities and solutions to achieve agreed goals.

It also involves monitoring the success of projects, reviewing and evaluating outcomes and working to and within budgets. There is also the need to plan for contingencies. The skills for this aspect of the community work 'skills tool box' are under increasing pressure from employers and funders who want to see value for their resources. There are now a number of local-based short courses, often organized by university extramural departments and career services that offer opportunities for practitioners across a number of employment sectors to enhance their skills in planning and organizing. It is important that when community workers use this skill, they attempt to remain focused on their role of working *with* the community not *against* it.

Team working

The advantages of team working are well known, for example, it can aid problem solving and enable team members to accomplish bigger tasks as a group than if they were working as individuals. Similar to the theories and practice that inform group work, team working involves sharing the diversity of skills and knowledge that individuals bring to the setting. One of the hallmarks of good team working is clear and transparent communication between members. This avoids problems later in the project's work.

If handled well, team working can increase and improve relationships between team members in order to meet agreed goals. However, teams that are not well handled can prove to be damaging for the individuals concerned, for example, where trust breaks down or the lack of openness prevents sufficient communication taking place. The key, therefore, is team building which should involve both work-related activity and allocated social time with each other. There are numerous team-building activities that involve games and activities as well as using workshops, seminars and the employment of team training practitioners.

It is recognized, however, that a number of community workers are not employed in teams but instead work independently. They may, however, be using team building activities and techniques in the communities that they are engaged with and the above will be of relevance to them.

Research skills

Undertaking research is crucial for effective community work. Research is a broad term but it is basically a systematic study of particular phenomena, a topic or in the case of community work, the study of a community or neighbourhood in order to ascertain the needs of the community or neighbourhood. Whether it is collecting information on a localized level, undertaking a community profile, writing a paper, article or piece for publication, they all require research skills. The reason why it is crucial is that, without the collection of information or research, the activity of community work is limited. During the 1970s and 1980s a well-used slogan in community work was 'information is power', and Saul Alinsky clearly demonstrated in the USA that if a community group or a campaign has pertinent information, it is in a strong position to be able to tackle even the largest of corporations and public authorities with both cogent arguments and focused action.

There are two main forms of research, both of which are valuable for community work: primary research which generates new information or data; and secondary research which uses existing data for a new purpose. In addition to these main forms of research one can add qualitative research methods and quantitative research methods. Qualitative research is a useful method for community work, as it involves the collection of descriptive information usually through questioning or observation. There is no one single qualitative method, rather, a number of alternative often flexible methods. One such example is ethnography which can involve studying a particular group or community by living or working with the people concerned in order to collect information on their lifestyles, beliefs, values, and so on.

Quantitative research methods use statistics in order to produce a description or analysis of a situation. This method has been used in the natural and health sciences where the researcher is interested in numerical frequencies.

While research skills are important for community work, few books have been written in the area. Among the exceptions is a helpful edited text by Mayo et al. (2013) that focuses on the role that research can play to assist in strengthening community development and working towards social justice and promoting active citizenship in the UK. Another useful, well-written, practically focused text is that by Stoecker (2013) that provides readers with guidance on how to use a project-based research model in the community. Finally, an edited text on how community research can be used with and for different communities with contributions from across the globe is Goodson and Phillimore (2012).

Community work skills: 'neutral' or political?

There has been some debate as to whether community work skills are 'neutral' and can be seen only as technical tools that can be deployed by anyone and whatever their ideology or values. Alternatively, does the community worker need to have particular values to successfully use these skills?

For the answer we need to return to the value base of community work which clearly indicates where the activity sits in the process of challenging power and offering alternatives. This, together with its creative aspect, is what makes community work a unique and important activity in the enhancement of democracy and the civil society.

Robertson (1991) warns that skills are not 'neutral' tools and expresses the belief that community workers need to be clear about their own and others' values before practising these skills. On the same tack, Dominelli (2006) argues that social problems need to be redefined in order to acknowledge the power relations that permeate society, particularly those between men and women, and between black and white people. This, she argues, can lead to developing and practising specific skills, as well as sharing skills. Dominelli (2006) identified the problems addressed by feminists and the skills needed to implement a successful campaign. She therefore interprets existing skills and demonstrates how they can be used by feminists. For instance, she highlights handling the media as a skill area, and discusses how female community workers can deal with the media that attempt to incorporate, sensationalize and ridicule those striving to communicate an alternative or radical viewpoint. Similarly, Dominelli argues that creating 'networks is a crucial ingredient in facilitating the processes whereby women make contact with and secure support from other women' (2006: 116).

In Chapter 7 we noted the influence of Freire's writings on the community work literature and in practice. The theory and practice presented by this adult educator have been interpreted by a number of practitioners and writers, with Ledwith (2011) providing one of the most comprehensive accounts of the impact of Freire on her ideas and practice and those of others. Sister Doreen Grant, working in the Govan district in Glasgow, also highlights the influence of Freire in her practice, when she points to the importance of the skills of co-operation, co-ordination and dialogue (Grant 1989). Based on their experiences of community work also in Glasgow, Bryant and Bryant (1982) identify the following skills for a 'good community worker': relationship skills; communication skills; organizational skills; mediating skills; negotiating skills; entrepreneurial skills; research skills; political and analytical skills; and tactical skills. The work and writings of Grant and Bryant and Bryant claim to be rooted in experiences of working-class communities and areas of economic and social deprivation. This leads the writers to state that community workers need to recognize that skills by themselves are insufficient to overcome major structural inequality. However, there is in such communities 'creative scope for helping to unleash capacities for self-organization and political expression amongst citizens who have been previously excluded from the public life of their city' (Bryant and Bryant 1982: 26).

In response to our question as to whether community work skills are neutral or political, we can see that while skills are transferable and can be used by practitioners from different ideological perspectives, it can also be argued that skills are not 'neutral' but have to be placed alongside and used in tandem with an understanding of the structural inequalities in society.

However, as we have noted throughout our discussions, the focus at the level of the locality has been considered by a number of writers to offer a narrow and an incomplete focus. We have also discovered that a more substantial understanding is available to us if it is recognized that both communities and community work can reflect the class, gender, and racially structured nature of society that distributes power and resources in an inequitable manner. We can further propose, therefore, that for those who believe community work is concerned with challenging societal inequalities, the skills it employs have to be adapted and re-created to address these.

Community work education and training

The UK community work education and training scene is relatively diverse and can be divided into full-time and part-time college-based courses; and a wide variety of field-based and employer-led programmes.

Over the years there has been concern to provide a co-ordinated and agreed standard of appropriate training for the diverse range of people who undertake or wish to undertake community work thus requiring an equally diverse range of accessible education and training opportunities. There have been numerous attempts to achieve a universal agreement on the skills and knowledge needed to produce competent community work programmes but to date that has not been achieved, though there has been some progress in the field of UK community development where the Federation for Community Development Learning has developed national occupational standards (see www.fcdl.org.uk/NOS). Although there is a lack of commonality between the various routes, with a diversity of material taught, and different bodies and universities validating the awards, none of which has community work as its main or only focus, the National Youth Agency has played a major role in professionally validating programmes.

To qualify as a community worker, it is necessary to undertake a college-based community work education course in one of a range of full-time and part-time programmes at post-graduate, post-qualifying, and initial training level and which include community work theory and practice as a constituent part of a wider study base.

As we noted in Chapter 3 when we discussed the development of community work, the activity has been associated with youth work since the late 1960s. It was in the aftermath of the Fairbairn-Milson Report (DES 1969) that existing youth work training courses retitled themselves 'youth and community work' training courses (Jeffs 1979: 61). This 'set youth work within the context of community development and its contribution towards a more participatory democracy' (Thomas 1983: 27).

The Conservative governments of the 1980s and 1990s, through the Department of Education and Science and later the Department for Education, were keen to emphasize youth work at the expense of community work, both on training courses and in the delivery of local authority youth services. This was because many of the traditional youth work posts that related to the management and administration of purpose-built youth clubs were difficult to fill. Instead, many graduates from youth and community work courses preferred employment in community work rather than youth work, or chose to work in other 'people-work professions' such as social work (Kuper 1985). The move to youth work rather than youth and community work was also influenced by the government's belief that youth workers had a role in providing activities and support to unemployed young people (Spence 1985; Williamson 1988).

At the time of writing there are 25 undergraduate courses in the UK where community work is in the title of the programme offered. Similarly there are ten universities offering 11 postgraduate diploma and master's community work courses, nearly all of which are linked to youth work. Although there is a wide and varying curriculum for these programmes, all are aimed at developing the skills and knowledge needed for work in the public sector, including local government housing and regeneration departments, education, leisure and social services departments, and the voluntary sector. The diversity of the programmes means there are opportunities for students to specialize in particular areas of community work, for example, work with women, engagement with ethnic minorities, anti-racist work, and community leadership and management. Programmes offer placements in various community-based agencies in order for students to develop their skill levels with individuals and groups and to further increase and deepen their understanding of social structures, processes and change. Experiences in placements together with learning at the university also provide students with the opportunity to reflect on their developing value base. Most programmes require students to undertake an extended piece of research through a supervised dissertation. This increases their research-mindedness and underlines the importance of developing research skills.

The part-time nature of these courses has significantly developed in recent years with many programmes designed to enhance professional practice and to advance processes aimed at inter-professional learning and working. Some students on these part-time programmes are supported by their employers who expect the practical module of the course to be located in the agency.

As referred to above, the National Youth Agency professionally validates degree, graduate certificate certificates and postgraduate diplomas and master's programmes that are monitored annually and where youth work is a major and constituent element. As we have seen, these programmes can also include community work as a component and this is one way for those who wish to practise community work on graduation to receive professional recognition.

There are also a number of local field-based and employer-led opportunities for community workers, and details on these many and varied schemes including one-day workshops and specific skill-based development can be accessed through organizations such as the Federation for Community Learning (www.fcdl.org.uk) and Lifelong Learning UK (www.lluk.org).

The employment of community workers

In 2007, the Community Development Foundation estimated something in the region of 20,000 community workers were engaged in the activity (CDF 2007). However, to reveal more detail on the employment of community workers we can turn to two in-depth surveys: the report by Glen et al. (2004), and the work by Sender et al. (2010).

Examining first the Glen et al. (2004) report, the research of which focused on community development workers and was managed by the Standing Conference for Community Development (SCCD) and the Community Development Foundation (CDF), we discover some important themes. Surveying community development workers took place in 2002 through a postal survey, of which 2,866 questionnaires were completed; regional workshops with practitioners which were held before the survey was launched in order to shape the survey questions and towards the end of the research to capture feedback on the initial analysis; and a study of unpaid workers in two locations. The research found that:

- The main source of funding for the posts surveyed was from the government with local government funding 35 per cent of posts and central government funding 27 per cent of posts. European funding covered 8 per cent of jobs, and charitable funds and the Community Fund financing 19 per cent of posts.
- A degree of instability and casualization was noticeable in the profession. The study found that since the 1980s there had been an erosion of permanent posts in the field and a similar increase in short-term contracts with some 39 per cent employed in such a capacity.
- Female practitioners were more likely to be employed on shorter contracts and almost twice as likely to be in part-time employment.

Women were also more likely than men to be on a lower pay scale. Further, the study found that community development is not a well-paid job, with over 70 per cent of workers on pay scales below £25,000 full-time equivalent, with only 6 per cent earning more than £30,000 per year. It was found that part-time workers were three times more likely than full-time workers to earn less than £16,000 full-time equivalent.

- The qualifications and experience required for a community work post varied and many practitioners were voicing concern that they found it difficult to access relevant training and obtain appropriate supervision. Barriers to accessing training included time restraints and lack of funds. In relation to support and supervision the survey found that 78 per cent of workers said their supervision was actually line management with 25 per cent of respondents saying their supervisors had no experience in the field. We will be looking at this factor in the section below on community work management.
- A number of unpaid workers were undertaking roles previously considered to be suitable for professional workers.
- Just over half (53 per cent) of the 2,866 respondents were employed in the voluntary sector while 42 per cent were employed in the statutory sector. Eight per cent were employed by 'partnerships' and 1 per cent in the private sector.

Overall, these findings are worrying as they show that community work, and in the case here specifically community development, although regarded as a valued activity, is prone to changes in wider government policy. So while community work provides a much-needed voice for those in communities, it is often a victim of financial cuts by governments that are suspicious and critical of an activity that can oppose their policies.

The more recent *Report of a Survey of Community Development Practitioners and Managers* (Sender et al. 2010) involved a smaller number of respondents (901) undertaking an online survey in 2009. All the respondents were based in England and the results provided valuable findings which included:

- Concerns relating to the impact of the 2008–09 recession and the resultant funding cuts. Like the Glen et al. (2004) survey, it noted that short-term funding was experienced as a major challenge with smaller organizations losing out to larger charities.
- Community development has an ageing workforce. The majority of survey respondents were women and over the age of 44, with male respondents likely to be older. The percentage of respondents over the age of 44 had increased to 62 per cent compared with 37 per cent in the earlier Glen et al. (2004) survey.

- The number of disabled respondents mirrored the proportion of disabled people in England as per the 2001 census. Slightly over a fifth of respondents were from black, Asian and minority backgrounds, which is higher than that reflected in the census.
- The most common employer for paid community development workers was the voluntary and community sector, with local authorities second.
- Most practitioners were earning between £20,000 and £30,000 with managers on salaries of between £25,000 and £35,000.
- Volunteers play an important role in community development but many expressed the view they did not receive sufficient support for undertaking their contribution.

Like the Glen et al. (2004) report, this Community Development Foundation report provides us with a valuable picture of the activity and the challenges faced by practitioners, managers and volunteers. In particular, the report confirms the diversity of the work undertaken and the types of agencies employing practitioners. Again similar to the earlier report, there can be little doubt that the activity has an important role to play in civic society and in particular in the bridging function between communities and the state, but it remains vulnerable to funding cuts and changes in social, economic and political policy.

Community work management

As we have already noted, a central concern for much of community work practice is the achievement of a more meaningful management of the resources available in a particular community or neighbourhood. This can include the management of staff. However, the extent to which this can and does happen is far from clear and such a commitment can be contentious.

One of the problems we find when examining the management of community work is the paucity of material on which to make observations and assessments. Arguably this is due in the main to the reticence felt by community workers about some of the central concepts of management, which have often been associated with hierarchical and elitist structures and run counter to activities concerned with participation and the devolution of power. This situation is not helped by the increasing pressure brought about by the implementation in public bodies of new managerialism.

In Chapter 1 we briefly referred to new managerialism and how it has had a negative impact on the public sector. This managerialist-driven practice is also termed New Public Management (NPM) which is often linked with the concept of evidence-based practice (EBP). EBP, which had its origins in science and medicine, is the presumption that interventions should be based on what is proven to work. The idea behind this is that this is likely to be cost-effective and with a predictable outcome. However, in community work this is far from certain to be successful, as individuals and communities are so variable. The concern too is that EBP can be used to focus on the outcomes produced by the practitioner and be a way of assessing their performance. However, in its defence, Chanan (2003) argues that evidence has been valuable in demonstrating that the establishing of social capital is a precondition for the accomplishment of successful neighbourhood regeneration programmes.

NPM has been described as:

> a shift by public sector leaders from policy to management; interest in quantifiable performance measures and appraisal; the break-up of structures into business units purchasing services from one another; market testing and tendering, rather than automatic in-house service provision; an emphasis on cost-cutting, output targets, rather than input controls; short-term contracts for staff, rather than 'jobs for life'; and the use of regulatory mechanisms, rather than legislation to ensure quality.
>
> (Turbett 2014: 16)

Despite the imposition of NPM as a method of managing community work, practitioners are recognizing that, serious reservations notwithstanding, as a way of managing services this approach is likely to be around in the public sector for the foreseeable future. Nevertheless the report by Sender et al. (2010), referred to in the previous section, recommends that employers should minimize the bureaucratic burdens on practitioners who in the 2009 survey were saying they wanted to spend up to another 12 per cent of their time working directly with communities rather than having to undertake tasks demanded by managers.

One publication that does provide community workers with a guide to a range of models and practices for the management of their work is Banks et al. (2013). This broad edited text discusses the challenges of engaging with communities where the involvement of citizens is to be encouraged, and yet the practitioners themselves are managed in ways which are counter to these values. This is well presented in the contribution by Mayo and Robertson who state:

> If managers of community practice and practitioners are seriously committed to making a difference, stretching the potential of the programmes that they work on to the limits, then they do need to develop a strategic approach based upon a clear understanding of

their opportunities, rooted in a critical analysis of the structural and policy constraints. This involves unpacking the contested concepts and the policy competing agendas . . . A commitment to working in more empowering ways, as reflective practitioners, rooted in the values of equal opportunities and social justice, involves developing strategies in partnerships with others.

(Mayo and Robertson 2013: 44)

What does the managing of community resources involve? Marilyn Taylor, who has written widely on the subject, offers a helpful list of tasks which includes 'financial control, policy, fundraising, political protection, hiring and firing, administration, accountability, advice and support to staff, monitoring and evaluation' (Taylor 1979: 2). Another writer in the area identifies a number of themes that involve management skills and knowledge, including the management of agencies and projects; the management of budgets; the management of change; the management of difficult and testing situations; local management; the management of people; the management of performance; the management of recruitment; the management of team building; and the management of volunteers (Twelvetrees 2008).

It is clear then that management of community work is a complex area and can cover many different and important strands that practitioners, employing organizations and agencies have to deal with every day. This wide remit for management is linked to the diversity of community work and the different forms of management that are needed to oversee the work undertaken. These range from the majority of UK local authorities which have developed NPM, and the minority that have pursued forms of decentralization, to community work projects and organizations that have *ad hoc* committees or support groups rooted in specific neighbourhoods or localities.

The management of community work ultimately involves accountability and control. If that management takes place within a hierarchical structure, as local authority community work does, and that activity is a marginal one, then there are certain implications for the practice. This makes the work of the practitioners challenging and requires them to work in ways that demand that they hold true to their role to assist the process of supporting people in the improvement of their communities. This means they need to collaborate where necessary with locally elected representatives and other key practitioners, as well as always working alongside the community itself in developing policies and processes that meet the objectives of both those who fund the activity, those who are engaged in it, and those who are its primary targets.

Community workers employed and managed in local authority departments are often but not always a constituent part of a team, which is in contrast to the situation in the 1970s where workers were often working in isolation (Thomas 1983: 229). There is a need, however, that as community workers progress in their work and increasingly take on more tasks involving management skills and knowledge, they will require further training and support. This training requirement is to some extent being met by the part-time programmes based in colleges and universities that were referred to above. It also means that practitioners should be encouraged and supported to attend training events, both in-house and those provided by external bodies and trainers.

In conclusion in this discussion of local authority community work, we can refer to the research undertaken some years ago now by Barr (1991), in which he reveals the overwhelming response from the community workers interviewed was that their managers wished to impose unnecessary limitations on their work. Further, they felt that their status was considered second-class relative to their social work colleagues. In response, Barr questions whether community work should be located in a department such as social services. He concludes by stating that if local authorities are serious in their commitment to community work, they should manage the activity in a manner that

> is consistent with empowering and enabling community organisations to participate and have influence ... Anything less than this promotes contradictions in behaviour of different categories of worker and legitimates allegations that community work is a token gesture, a sop to the notion of consumer sovereignty.
>
> (Barr 1991: 82)

Community work that is funded at least in part by the state and is delivered through the work of voluntary agencies has different management styles and procedures. Historically, the ability to manage community work in more varied ways is greater in the voluntary sector than in the local authority sector, because this is not subject to the pressures that we have discussed above. This has led to a range of different styles of management, including self-management or collective working and management (Stanton 1989), and structureless or leaderless groups and management (Freeman 1984). However, as we have previously noted, the financing and control of community work have changed in recent years. This has influenced the management of the activity within the voluntary and charitable sector. The greater scrutiny by the state of its funding and the desire to influence and direct the development of community work, have led central and local government to encourage the major voluntary organizations that it funds to concentrate a proportion of their resources in assisting in the development of management training. For instance, the National Council for Voluntary Organisations has taken a prominent role in attempting to improve the management of community work through a range of publications and training events (www.ncvo.org.uk). Similarly the National Youth Agency has tackled the issue through similar means (www.nya.org.uk), as have the Community Development Foundation (http://cdf.org.uk). The Federation for Community Development Learning (www.fcdl.org.uk), which is a UK-wide network, has as one of its roles the training in this area.

These organizations and a number of their management publications make a point of emphasizing that attracting state funding is becoming more difficult and that voluntary organizations which have clear objectives and well-defined management structures are more likely to be in receipt of this declining finance.

Another important issue in the management of community work in the voluntary sector is the role of the principal manager of small voluntary agencies. Peatfield (1992) made a study of eight voluntary agencies, all of them employing a 'director', 'co-ordinator' or 'organizer', who is responsible to a voluntary committee for the management of the work of a small staff team. Peatfield found that all the managers surveyed suffered a great deal of stress, often related to their complex and ambiguous role and to the small amount of supervision and support they received in their work. The research discovered that in the absence of leadership from their committees, the managers assumed the burden of providing their agencies with a sense of direction, often acting as interpreters of unclear policies and procedures. They also frequently had to cope with a wide range of different and often irreconcilable tasks. Peatfield found that managers brought to the position individual 'packages' of interests and experience and considerable commitment to the agency. All those he interviewed had succeeded in developing their own system for ensuring that the work was undertaken successfully. The author suggests that these managers can be seen as successful 'voluntary sector entrepreneurs', whose approach resembles that of a small business owner. However, this success has been achieved at a cost. Peatfield found that managers feel indispensable and are unable to sustain the effort for long periods. This can lead to agencies losing a sense of collective purpose and experiencing difficulties when their manager decides to resign. As a long-term solution, Peatfield suggests that the performance of management committees could be improved. In the meantime, the author argues, agencies should reduce the range of tasks they expect their managers to tackle, and provide them with more systematic induction, supervision and support.

Conclusion

In this chapter we have discussed a number of central themes in community work practice. We have noted that values are central to community work and are related to addressing the implications of structural and personal inequality and disadvantage. We also are aware that while the protection of democracy is a fundamental value in society, we are conscious that the present representative democracy fails to properly reflect the many issues that concern the public. Hence the need for a strong and active civil society in which community work can play a role.

Our discussion on community work skills highlighted the many different skills that practitioners need on order to undertake their work. We also identified seven skills that a community worker will want in their 'skills tool box' to practise effectively. Importantly we were able to state that skills are not neutral but instead have to be placed alongside our values and our understanding of the inequalities and discrimination that make up our society.

Community work education and training are fundamental to improving and extending the practice of the activity. In the UK community work education and training is diverse and to some extent fragmented. However, it is crucial that this work receives constant attention and support in order that it is able to thrive.

The surveys on community development have provided us with a valuable snapshot of the activity as seen by practitioners, managers and unpaid volunteers. Both surveys referred to confirm the potentially fragile nature of the activity in terms of funding and yet it is recognized to be carrying out a vital role in advancing civic society.

Finally, we discussed the importance of appropriate management styles for community work. This is in the face of new managerialism or NPM which has a value system at odds with those in community work.

Part of the difficulty we experience when examining much of the above work is the lack of satisfactory research into aspects of community work practice. Although there are a number of specific surveys and reports on community work practice, many of these are now dated and often not comprehensive. This gap in the literature has not assisted the development of a coherent theory and practice of community work. We can speculate on the reasons for this gap. One could be the diverse and often ambiguous meanings given to community work. A clearer idea of what comprises community work could assist in the recognition of its areas of practice. Similarly, more research on practice that produces data and evidence could enhance the activity's development. At the present time there are a number of organizations and individuals that do contribute to researching practice and their work has been drawn upon in this chapter. There is, however, a clear need to raise the research profile in community work if we are to appreciate the changes the activity is facing and the development it can make. The results of such endeavours will enable community work to argue more effectively for the scarce resources available in the public sector.

Questions

1 Identify your personal values and how they are enacted in your practice.
2 Consider how you would rate the skills needed for effective community work practice on a scale of 1–5, with 1 being the least important and 5 being the most important. Explain the reasons for your decisions.

9 Community work internationally

Community work is an internationally recognized activity that is as diverse as the countries where it is practised. This edition of *Analysing Community Work* has focused on developments in the UK at the same time as making reference to and connections with community work in other parts of the world.

While the concept of community work internationally has been used to describe a range of different understandings of practice and outcomes, in all cases it is concerned with improving the lives of individuals and groups in designated areas, communities or geographical localities, and it is nearly always seeking solutions to and working with people experiencing poverty, disadvantage and discrimination. Community work internationally is similar to that in the UK in that it can range from well-resourced state-sponsored programmes to localized and independent projects that usually rely on the energy and commitment of a small number of people and have at their disposal few material resources. However, the success of community work anywhere depends on harnessing the skills, knowledge and vision of those who are committed to addressing the shared concerns and key issues that impact on localities and communities of interest.

In this chapter we will start by considering the work of two leading international organizations, one of which publishes a peer-reviewed journal, *Community Development: Journal of the Community Development Society*, before reviewing the influential *Community Development Journal*. These organizations and their activities have had a significant impact on community work world-wide and in particular in the area of community development.

We then refer to the work of Beck and Purcell (2013), followed by a consideration of global citizen action, both of which provide us with a further critical understanding of community work internationally. After this, we consider the work of one particular community work project in Hong Kong, which is working with local residents to challenge the impact of neo-liberal policies and practices. Finally, the chapter ends with a call for community work to consolidate its international links so that the patchwork of activity is more than just that.

The International Association for Community Development (IACD)

Arguably the most influential community work world-wide organization is the not-for-profit, non-government membership International Association for Community Development (IACD) which 'is a global network of community development organisations, practitioners, researchers, activists and policy makers who are committed to issues of global justice' (IACD 2013: 2). While the administrative centre is based in Scotland, the IACD is an organization with almost 500 members in 46 countries and has an international Board of Directors, each representing one of seven global regions. This well connected dynamic organization relies on the energies and commitment of its global membership in order to sustain its numerous activities and contribute to its many publications, local forums, international conferences, events, gatherings, blogs, podcasts, videos and its increasing presence on social media. The main purpose of these various activities is to enable members to share knowledge and learning in order to enrich and sustain community development practice and policy internationally. Further, the activities provide individual IACD members with a shared sense of connectedness across vast geographical regions as well as across the globe.

One of the recurring issues for sustaining the future of the IACD has been to ensure it has sufficient funding in order to maintain its presence in the community development field and to keep alive its many different activities. The organization depends on contributions from grant funders, donations and legacies, membership fees and contributions, together with fee income and other charges to finance the administration of the organization, the principal cost being that of staff, and to support events and developments. IACD members and supporters give their time free of charge and usually make a significant personal financial contribution to their travel to events and inter-national conferences. Without this it is highly unlikely the organization would survive. Further details on IACD, including details of its events, publications and resources can be accessed on www.iacdglobal.org.

The Community Development Society (CDS)

The Community Development Society (CDS) is a USA-based organization with almost 80 per cent of its members practising there and another 20 per cent working in 32 different countries. The CDS members work in a range of sectors, including education, health care, social services, government, and economic development. The Society's peer-reviewed journal, the *Community Development: Journal of the Community Development Society* is published five times a year and focuses on disseminating information on theory, research and practice with articles covering such diverse topics as rural and urban economic development, housing, entrepreneurship, theory, technology, social capital, and leadership.

As well as hosting local events, the CDS international annual conference provides an opportunity for members to meet and to renew networks with community development practitioners, academics and policy-makers based both in the USA and internationally, while debating particular developments in the field. The Society makes a number of awards each year to recognize high-quality and innovative practice among its members. Further information on the CDS can be accessed at www.comm-dev.org

The *Community Development Journal*

First published in 1966, the *Community Development Journal* (CDJ) has occupied an important place in the development of community work internationally. Published four times a year and considered to be the leading journal in its field, the CDJ has almost 1,000 subscribers in over 80 countries, with many more readers accessing it online and through library copies.

The principal activity of the CDJ has been to increase the understanding of the theory and practice of community development internationally, and the Editorial Board, though it is drawn almost completely from the UK, has worked tirelessly to produce a journal that is truly global in its scope and contents:

> The Board, aware it could be criticised for being primarily UK based, put in a good deal of energy into the Special Issues that had an international content. Guest editors were located and invited to produce a selection of special issues on subjects as diverse as community development and social movements; livestock and community development; women, poverty and community development; and Latin America.
>
> (Popple 2003: 212)

A text that provides a representative sample of the best writing in the CDJ since its first publication in 1966 is Craig et al. (2008). Thirty articles were selected by the three book editors, two of whom are former editors of the journal, to demonstrate the richness and diversity of community development theory and practice internationally. The edited volume has a particularly helpful introductory chapter by Mayo (2008) which provides a historical context for the advance of community development over almost five decades and as reflected in the selected articles. Focusing on the lessons that can be learnt from the articles from around the globe, Mayo (2008: 26) states;

> Perhaps the key lesson may be the lesson that has already been drawn – the lesson about the importance of strategic thinking, in the face of increasing complexity, strategic thinking about perspectives and long-term goals and strategic thinking about ways of identifying the spaces for creative practice in the context of globalisation. Global advocacy and campaigning would seem to be most effective when soundly rooted in local constituencies, communities, trade union organisations and their allies in civil society, relating global issues to local priorities.

The CDJ continues to adopt a broad definition of community development to include aspects such as policy, planning and action, publishing papers that raise questions of social justice, diversity and environmental sustainability. Published since its launch by the Oxford University Press, the journal is financially stable, has organized occasional conferences, and published working papers, and with its committed and energetic Editorial Board and an International Advisory Board, it is likely to be in existence for many years to come. Further information on the CDJ can be found at www.cdj.oxfordjournals.org

Community organizing internationally

For readers who want to specifically consider community organizing internationally in more depth, the text by Beck and Purcell (2013), together with various articles in the above-mentioned two journals will prove useful. The work by Beck and Purcell (2013) explores the diversity of the practice in six different countries: the USA, the UK, India, South Africa, Cambodia and Australia. In particular, Beck and Purcell examine the legacy of the practice and ideas of Saul Alinsky, with the authors stating that 'the experience and the opportunities of poor people around the world are greatly enhanced if they are organised' (2013: 18). One of the key features of the book is the analysis of the lessons that can be learnt from the developments in community organizing across the globe as well as helping us to recognize the similarities and differences that the activity has in both the Global North and the Global South.

Based on their extensive fieldwork which included questionnaires and visits to projects in the six countries, the authors argue that, while community organizing is [strong] in terms of its tactics, identification of local issues and mobil-ising people for change. We think it is less strong in the development of critical thinking and reflection on the one hand, and citing its prac-tice within broader political thinking and political movements on the other.

(Beck and Purcell 2013: 177)

This is an important finding and one we will be returning to later in this chapter and in the final chapter.

Global citizen action

One of the benefits of considering community work internationally is the links that can be made across the globe at a local level to challenge the damage inflicted by a neo-liberal globalizing world. An important challenge for community work which has been a theme of this second edition is to consider moving away from the 'think globally, act locally' mantra to one where we need to consider locally how the global institutions, corporations and forces are impacting on our communities. In what way are our daily lives affected by the practice of these enormous financial organizations and banks, powerful global media organizations like that controlled by the Murdoch family, massive retail industries such as Wal-Mart and Primark, many of which exploit labour in the Global South to sell goods cheaply in the Global North, and world trade organizations like the WTO and the IMF that sanction and encourage this approach to trade? By pursuing this line of thought, our local practice then connects with the analysis of the wider changing and unequal power structures, while helping us make connections with struggles with groups and people throughout the world.

Although the literature in the field of connecting the impact of these major forces on local communities is still developing, the reader is alerted to the edited text by Edwards and Gaventa (2001) in which the authors highlight the need for 'building from the bottom up'. To quote the editors:

By laying a strong foundation for negotiations over labor standards, environmental pollution, and human rights, they offer the potential to connect ordinary citizens to global regimes. But this can only work if local structures are connected to more democratic structures at higher levels of the world system, which can ensure that the sacrifices made in one location are not exploited by less scrupulous counterparts elsewhere.

(Edwards and Gaventa 2001: 8)

One of the features of global citizen action has been the large public protests that have occurred that connect people across the globe with each other. In the last 20 years there have been a number of high profile struggles and campaigns both globally and more localized that have focused on the impact of multinational corporations and bodies. Perhaps the best-known of these protests is that which took place on 30 November 1999 in Seattle, Washington State, USA, where the World Trade Organization ministerial conference was launching its trade negotiations. Local, regional, national and international groups and NGOs, especially those concerned with environmental, consumer and labour rights and issues, numbering some 40,000 in total, planned and attended a large protest outside the Washington State Trade and Convention Center. This brought together a number of strands of protest with unions and consumer protection groups concerned about competition of unsafe imports, products made by cheap foreign labour, environmentalists focusing on the outsourcing of polluting activities, labour rights groups protesting about bad working conditions in other countries, and radical and Left groups concerned with the power of globalizing capitalism. This landmark protest was known too for the high level of policing and the use of equipment such as rubber bullets and tear gas in response to the protestors.

Pokfulam Village: a community work project to sustain a heritage settlement

Hong Kong Island is home to Pokfulam Village which is believed to have been established in the early part of the eighteenth century. Over the years the village has been transformed from a simple agricultural community to a residential community. It has in its time been a local commercial centre and during the 1950s provided a variety of services to the surrounding area as well as being the location of a thriving dairy farm. During the period 1940–80, the village underwent a regeneration and many of the houses were built of material by Chinese refugees, which are now considered to be shabby and out of place with the luxury villas that are being built close by.

With a population of around 3,000, 15 per cent of the residents of Pokfulam Village are over the age of 65, while 20 per cent are under 18 years. The housing profile is a mixture of private tenants and owner occupiers.

Despite having been in existence for three centuries, the village is under threat from developers who are keen to buy this rare 4-acre site in order to build and sell luxury accommodation. Half of the land on which the village is located is privately owned by the original clans who have settled there over the past three centuries, and the other half is owned by various licensees and the Hong Kong government. One of the key issues for the local community is that all temporary structures built on government land are regulated under a squatter control policy. This policy restricts the use of material and the size of structures that can be built there. It has meant that residents' property is deteriorating and with the impending threat of clearance of the area, people have not been investing in their homes and previously were reluctant to engage in environment management.

It is against this background that the Caritas Pokfulam Community Development Project is operating. Established and funded by the Hong Kong Catholic Church, the project now receives significant support from the Hong Kong government. However, according to local community workers, the funding of projects is not secure as the government has a reputation for closing down troublesome community work organizations. Nevertheless the Caritas Pokfulam Community Development Project practitioners have been working closely with the residents and together have made a considerable impact, so much so that in 2014 the village gained international recognition for its struggle and was listed on the World Monuments Watch List by the New York-based World Monuments Fund. The listing by the Fund, whose aim is to protect monuments (including villages such as Pokfulam) and is able to provide professional support and resources for projects, led the Hong Kong government to send senior officials and elected representatives to the village to listen to the residents' wish to see the area become a sustainable settlement through legislation.

A central theme of the community work project has been to organize a number of art workshops and festivals; setting up art installations and photographic shows; the formation of a credit union; and the creation of a communal garden to cultivate vegetables that can be shared among fellow villagers. The community workers have run workshops on food recycling, and sessions on reflecting on the use of domestic chemicals. The outcome of these workshops has led to residents creating a village compost area, the fertilizer from which has been used in the communal garden.

The drive to conserve the village and to revitalize community spirit has begun to transform the feelings of residents from having little hope (in 2011, a three-year mental health project found that slightly more than a third of the population suffered from depression) to one of feelings of success and the possibility that against the odds they can continue to live there, despite the pressure from developers who want to secure the land for private profit. Villagers meet on a regular basis with government officers to press for improvements in the neighbourhood, have provided guides to those who want to visit the traditional Hong Kong village and to see the steps it has made to sustain the heritage of the community while hearing how the residents have pressed for the upgrading of the basic infrastructure.

This short case study provides a valuable insight into a community work project that is operating in a neigbourhood that is experiencing the impact of neo-liberal economic policies. In fact, Hong Kong, which is an important centre for international trade and finance and with a cosmopolitan society, is a good example of the neo-liberal economic and social project. This Special

Administrative Area (SRA) of the People's Republic of China (China is some-times referred to as one country, two systems) is one of the most densely populated regions in the world, has one of the highest per capita incomes in the world, and has one of the highest income inequalities among advanced economies (Carroll 2007). As a consequence, land is at a premium and has had an impact on property prices throughout the SRA, hence the property developers putting pressure on the Hong Kong government to release the land in Pokfulam so that they can build high rise flats and villas. However, as we have seen, the local residents are working collectively together and in collab-oration with the other agencies to repel these possible developments and to build a more sustainable community that reflects their creative talents and their need to live in a harmonious neighbourhood that has a positive future.

Knitting together the global community work patchwork

One of the strengths of community work is its ability to work in difficult circum-stances to support individuals and groups in the most marginal urban and rural communities in order to give them a valid voice and to tackle the considerable pressures on them. As we have discussed in this chapter, two international organizations, the Community Development Society and the International Association of Community Development, have made great strides to link prac-titioners, academics, policy-makers and activists globally to make connections with each other and to share views and exchange understandings of practice. With the increasing use of technology and social media, this exchange can take place virtually as well as in person at conferences and events. These connec-tions are valuable at sharing the learning from experiences in group and campaign organizing, developing community leadership, enhancing skill devel-opment, and reflecting on the value base of community work.

One of the key roles that global community work organizations can play is working with the numerous disparate groups and individuals who are engaged in the activity to secure an overarching framework that nurtures and develops the shared values of the practice. Such organizations too are a place for contributing to the development of the theoretical base of community work that has been discussed in this book. This would assist in forming a cohesive basis to community work internationally which was also referred to by Beck and Purcell (2013).

Conclusion

Internationally, community work is in a positive state with examples given here of two organizations that are making an important contribution to strengthening the activity globally. Both these organizations arrange international and regional conferences and events that provide valuable opportunities for those involved in the work to network and to develop alliances. This supplements the numerous organizations and groups locally, regionally and nationally that provide support for the development of community work. Similarly, there are two well-established peer-review journals that provide a conduit for the regular dissemination of examples of practice, the results of research and developments in theoretical thinking.

We have also noted in this chapter the development of thinking and practice linked to global citizens action and to international community organization. The case study from Hong Kong provides us with an example of a project that is meeting the challenge of neo-liberal policies and land grab. Finally, we have discussed the importance of supporting and sustaining initiatives that are focused on strengthening community work globally.

Questions

1 Consider the impact of neo-liberal policies and of globalization on a community work project that you are familiar with. What responses can be made to the challenges that are presented?

2 How can you be involved in supporting community work internationally? Are you involved in an international organization or have you written for a community work journal that has an international readership? If not, is this something you could consider?

10 Conclusion and future directions

The second edition of *Analysing Community Work* has been written and published 20 years after the first edition was published. What started out as a project to make minor revisions to a much referred text has turned out to be a major re-write and re-consideration of the role of community work in the twenty-first century. The world has changed in powerful and important ways in the past 20 years, and if I were to produce a third edition of the book in another 20 years, I suspect the changes reflected on would be even greater and more extensive than those of the last two decades.

Many of the key themes of the past 20 years have been raised and discussed in the previous chapters and these will be referred to in this final chapter, together with other important developments that are impacting on the communities in which we live and work. We will also look at how it may be possible for community work to respond to these advances and, importantly, how we can continue to make community work responsive to the huge tasks ahead.

We will start this chapter by giving a recap of a number of the major points made in the previous chapters. This is not an exhaustive review and readers may find that certain elements of book resonate for them more than others. However, what is presented here are examples of the enormous changes in our societies and the role community work can play.

1   *Communities are significantly changing.* There is little doubt that communities at the neighbourhood, regional, national and international levels are developing in ways that are distinctly different from what they were in the 1990s. We are now confronted with powerful and what often feels unrelenting economic, political and social forces that are shaping communities everywhere. These major forces are impacting on both neighbourhoods and communities of interest and identity. The old is being replaced by the new which is usually presented by politicians and others as 'better' or 'progressive' but is often

contested by many as further evidence of the state's power and the increasing influence of massive corporations.

We have seen the development of technology which, in the case of CCTV, is considered to be valuable in identifying those engaged in criminal behaviour, while sophisticated technology has been used by states everywhere to increase their surveillance of its citizens and subjects through the monitoring of emails, texts and telephone conversations in order to scrutinize what feels like everyone while excluding those considered to be a threat. It feels at times as if elements of George Orwell's famous terrifying dystopian novel, *Nineteen Eighty-Four* (Orwell 2013) have been introduced into everyday contemporary reality. At the same time the emergence of flexible forms of social media has enabled groups and individuals to develop alliances to organize and oppose exploitive developments. As well as being used by protestors in the Arab Spring of December 2010 onwards and those caught up in the siege of Gaza during July and August of 2014, social media has also been deployed by those engaged in the Occupy Movements and groups co-ordinating protests against intrusions into community life, as in the case of groups confronting companies engaged in fracking for shale gas.

2   *Social and economic inequalities are increasing in the UK and in most countries in the world.* The impact of the neo-liberal policies and globalization has, as Mirowski (2013: 28) argues, 'sunk its roots into everyday life' with societies both polarizing and fragmenting. In particular, we are seeing the shrinking of state services and the unleashing of powerful market forces in almost all areas of welfare, health, education, housing and services for vulnerable people, including those with mental health needs, prisoners, the elderly, and poor and disadvantaged children and families. Neo-liberalism advocates the primacy of the market over the state, unless of course there is a need for the state to intervene to maintain the primacy of the market and protect the wealthy in society. The result of this ideology in a period of austerity has led to deep cuts in public services, including community work projects, with communities and individuals being told that they must take responsibility for their own welfare.

While the UK is the seventh richest country in the world, it is a country of significant and growing inequality. Evidence presented by Cooper et al. (2014) indicates that the income of the bottom 90 per cent increased by 27 per cent between 1993 and 2011, however, during the same period, incomes for the richest 0.1 per cent of the population increased by 101 per cent. This means that the incomes of the top 0.1 per cent have grown almost four times faster than for the bottom 90 per cent of the population.

Cooper et al. (2014) argue that once increases in the cost of living over the last ten years are factored in, then the real squeeze for the majority of those living in the UK becomes apparent, as does the divide between those at the top and the rest. Since 2003, 95 per cent of the British public have experienced a 12 per cent real terms drop in their disposable income, whilst the richest 5 per cent of the population have enjoyed a healthy rise in their income.

To put this in context, we know that an English Premier League footballer can earn as much in a week as a NHS nurse does in ten years. Chief Executive Officers of some of the largest UK companies now receive payments of millions of pounds a year whilst those who clean the offices where these highly paid executives work are earning the minimum hourly wage or, in some cases, less. Meanwhile the British Labour Party, which was formed in the early part of the twentieth century out of struggles to ensure that workers were protected from the ravages of capitalism, had while in government in 1998 a Secretary for Trade and Industry (Peter Mandelson, now Lord Mandelson) who claimed that the Labour government were 'intensely relaxed about people getting filthy rich' (quoted by Selbourne 2014).

It is against this background that community work is now practised. Certain communities, groups and individuals, both in the UK and globally, have been ruthlessly cast adrift as the restructuring of society carries on at speed, with the most wealthy accumulating riches that the poorest in society can only dream about as their living standards fall and their life chances are restricted.

3   *The historical development of community work reflects the tension between the forces of benevolent paternalism and community action.* This analysis remains a valuable way of understanding the role the activity presently occupies in an increasingly unequal society. We have also seen that the historical development of the UK has involved a struggle between those with power and who support the dominant relations that emerged from establishing a powerful empire, and who support the aristocracy, the established church, exploitative employers and a benevolent elite; and those without privileges and influence and have been pressing against those in power, often at considerable cost and sacrifice. For those working from below, this struggle is about giving a voice to the voiceless as well as trying to rectify the power imbalance that is endemic in our society.

Democratic states will constantly need to deploy forms of local-based interventions that are focused on engaging communities that are experiencing stress and disadvantage; failure to do so can leave politicians open to criticism that the state is letting down those who are its constituents. Important too, the state is conscious that the disadvantaged and disenfranchised can become further disillusioned and angry and take action that seeks to threaten the status quo. Intervening in localities and communities and making concessions to those living there are intended to pacify and placate as well as providing the state with further opportunities to exercise control and surveillance over the population. These local-based interventions frequently employ community workers and/or community work strategies and skills.

A reading of the political and economic circumstances of Western countries shows that the post-war settlement that involved state governments engaging in improving the living standards of those residing in their countries was broken in the late 1970s and early 1980s. In the UK this has been accompanied with growing ideological attacks on certain groups. These attacks are focused on arguments that the welfare state is too large and public expenditure too great and should be reined in. This takes place alongside hegemonic assaults on labour, the trade union movement and welfare recipients. In response, we have seen oppositional counter-hegemonic pressure in the form of local community action and national campaigns from those engaged in, and usually living in, particular communities that bear the brunt of the policies and practice of governments and corporations that privilege profit before people.

4 *New managerialism (or New Public Management) is the hand-maiden of neo-liberalism and its tentacles have penetrated the daily experience of community work.* In many cases, the professional discretion of community workers has been replaced by an emphasis on efficiency and productivity which can be overseen by managers with the use of technology. At the same time financial strategizing, hierarchical power structures and the managing of risk have been introduced into the public sector to define and measure specific outcomes. The introduction of routinized practices in organizations can lead to many of the complexities of people's daily lives not always being recognized by managers, meaning that community workers have to struggle to present their practice of empowerment in a manner that meets the demands that their work achieve certain targets and key performance indicators.

5 *The role of the civil society becomes ever more important at a time when parliamentary systems everywhere are under increasing pressure and when constituents have failing respect for politicians.* At the same time there is scepticism that politicians can effectively respond to the needs of voters. It is against this background that community work has a key role in strengthening civil society and offering counter-hegemonic ideas and practices. In most countries

the electoral process is under pressure, with elites demanding that their interests are placed before those of the majority of the population. Mainstream lobby groups, think tanks and economists are constantly attempting to influence governments to sustain the inequalities outlined above (Monbiot 2014). The justification of massive inequalities lies at the very centre of democracy, yet few politicians or political parties are heard championing the cause of those who suffer from the consequence of this race to cut taxes on capital and high incomes, of legalizing new tax avoidance schemes, while at the same time failing to invest sufficiently in much-needed public services. The building of community and social capital and the championing of community empowerment, however, is a keystone in the practice of community work. It is a way of bringing the needs of local communities to the forefront and of working to improve the life chances of those living in certain neighbourhoods and of members of specific groups. At the same time the practice of community work involves connecting with other organizations, cultural and social institutions, and different groupings, all of which can act as a counterbalance to the power of the state.

6   *The theories informing community work need to be constantly reviewed and analysed as to their value to the activity.* In the first edition of *Analysing Community Work*, emphasis was given to the importance of the work by Paulo Freire and Antonio Gramsci in assisting us in understanding both the macro-level forces operating in our society, and in considering how we can best intervene at the locality and community levels. The work of these two influential theoreticians and practitioners remains valuable. However, as demonstrated in Chapter 6, there are a number of other key thinkers and writers whose work can complement that of Freire and Gramsci and add to our developing understanding while providing us with ways of interpreting our practice and presenting methods of intervention that are valid.

7   *Over the past 20 years the evolution of the environmentalism and green movement critique has been an important theoretical and practice development and has much to offer community work.* As further evidence becomes available of the impact of man's degradation of the natural and social environment, and in particular the impact of the intensification of farming, industrial pollution, global warming and the depletion of the stocks of available resources, there are moves at the central and local state level to counter this with agreements to meet the United Nations Millennium Goals that include ensuring environmental sustainability.

Protection of the environment has also become a focus for a number of community-based groupings. The environmentalist and green movement critique, referred to in Chapters 6 and 7, is still in its infancy in its relationship to community work. However, arguably it has much to offer with its connections between local activism and protecting the environment globally.

8   *Values are at the heart of community work theory and practice and we have noted that the values of equality, social justice and anti-discrimination are three of the key values.* To these values we might want to add those of solidarity, collective action, democracy and a fundamental redistribution of wealth and power. These values stand in opposition to those of a society that is epitomized by ruthless competition, individualism, the supremacy of private profit and attacks on democracy by corporate and private interests.

The future of community work

Looking to the future of community work, we can see choppy seas ahead with continuing financial and service reductions in the public sector and a retrenchment from the values that established the welfare state. However, there is no reason why community work cannot continue the vital work it undertakes outside the direct remit of the state. Organizations like the global IACD, as well as more regional and national groupings, are examples of great enthusiasm and commitment to develop a community work practice that is relevant to the times in which we live.

Nevertheless there will always be a call for the state to address the needs of communities and groups affected by the economic and social turbulence of wide-scale significant change. Community work as presented in the models we have identified in Chapter 7 have a proven history of working effectively in neighbourhoods and local areas.

To enable community work to carry out this important project, it has to undertake a number of tasks, including continuing doing well what it is good at while moving into terrains that have not previously been considered as mainstream. For example, in a period of significant change in society with power being concentrated in the hands of the wealthy, the political elite and the major corporations, it is argued by some that community members can appear apathetic and lack engagement in the area in which they live. If this is the case, then it is likely to come as a response to the top-down political processes that leave residents little opportunity to properly engage in making meaningful decisions or feeding back their views to those who make choices on their behalf.

There is then a need to look outside of the usual community work approaches to how we interact with communities and to consider more seriously other ways of engaging with people. There are three such ways that community work could consider assisting in its engagement with communities, and in turn contributing to the development of the activity's theory and practice. These are: (1) the use of psycho-geography; (2) through a consideration of the benefits of collective narrative practice; and (3) by considering greater involvement in community economic development. These approaches are now presented.

Psycho-geography

One such approach that could assist the development of the theory and practice of community work is drawn from psycho-geography which emerged in the middle of the twentieth century as a form of understanding the nature and impact of urban spaces (Debord 1997). This approach emphasizes the impact of people's geography on their behaviour and emotions and arguably has lessons to offer community work as it explores how space shapes residents' views of themselves, their relationship to wider communities and their world-views. Importantly too the approach considers people's involvement in social and political aspects of the communities they engage with. In the UK, psycho-geography has largely been deployed in performance art and literature, for example, the writings of Peter Ackroyd (see, for example, Ackroyd 2001) and Iain Sinclair (see, for example, Sinclair 2003). Both these writers demonstrate how the hidden landscapes of atmospheres, histories, and actions can be used to describe and analyse urban spaces. The application of this method in community work resonates with the approaches advocated by Paulo Freire and the radical Brazilian theatre director and writer Augusto Boal (1931–2009) (see, for example, Boal 2008). Approaches informed by psycho-geography could arguably be used with groups so that people can re-examine their communities to renew their interest in and energy for the area in which they live and enjoy a greater appreciation of the neighbourhood. In turn, this could lead to an understanding of the challenges they face as community members and how they can best address these through community work.

Collective narrative practice

Another approach that can be used in community work is collective narrative practice, which has been developed by the Dulwich Centre in Adelaide, Australia, and who publish *The International Journal of Narrative Therapy and Community Work*. Based on the work of Paulo Freire, collective narrative practice is focused on listening and responding to the stories produced by individuals and groups, recognizing that while these stories represent personal experiences they also reflect and inform broader social issues. In particular, the approach is used with those experiencing hardship and trauma, and by acknowledging and encouraging the stories, it can help people reclaim their lives and tackle the harm and injustice done to them by engaging in personal and local social action.

The approach involves working with people to connect with local cultural mediums, including the written word, spoken word, song, film, dance, poetry and celebration. In this way people are able to perform, witness and share in ways that help them re-define their identity, and enable them to engage in ways which both provide relief from the effects of hardship and trauma *and* build personal and collective agency (Denborough 2008). Further information on collective narrative practice as developed by the Dulwich Centre is available at www.dulwichcentre.com.au/

Community economic development

We discussed this area of work in Chapter 7 when we were considering models of community work. Arguably, together with good health, the most important need for our populations is secure and adequate economic activity that can sustain people in useful and meaningful employment, and to provide financial support when needed. The drive for local economic development, often in opposition to the power of the multinationals, and which is democratic and socially just, would appear an important way forward for communities everywhere. Giving people more control over the economic sphere would provide a much needed lever to help people feel part of communities and neighbourhoods in which they live.

There are two other features of community work that need further development if the activity is to remain relevant for the coming years: research; and education and training.

Research and community work

At different stages in the book we have been made aware that there is a paucity of research which can assist us to better analyse community work. Nonetheless the situation has been improved in the past 20 years with key articles and commentaries published in the *Community Development Journal*, and the *Journal of the Community Development Society*. Similarly the International Association for Community Development, the Community Development Foundation, the Federation for Community Development Learning, as well as a number of other large and small organizations world-wide have done much to raise the profile of the activity and have produced material that has furthered the community work enterprise. Meanwhile community work texts, many of which have been referred to in this book, continue to play a valuable role in increasing the knowledge base for the activity. However, there is still much to be done to carry to a wider grouping the benefits of community work. A stronger research and publishing base will assist this process and explain why community work is important.

Education and training

The changes in university funding in the UK have had a detrimental impact on the education for community work at the higher education level. The introduction of university tuition fees of almost £10,000 per year for undergraduate degrees and significant fees for post-graduate courses and the subsequent reduction of those wanting to undertake community work programmes, which have uncertain employment opportunities for its graduates, has made many relevant courses uneconomic and they have since been closed. This has made it even more important to protect those programmes that still exist and to encourage the development of courses elsewhere.

In recent times I have been closely involved in the community work programmes at the National University of Ireland Maynooth, which has a portfolio of community work education programmes, ranging from those at undergraduate degree level to doctoral studies. These programmes provide students, who come from an array of backgrounds and reflect the diversity of the activity, with a stimulating and challenging environment to reflect on their practice and to develop further theoretical understandings that advance and enhance their action in the field. These programmes which offer recognized and endorsed qualifications are tailored to provide students with an in-depth understanding of the changing local, national and international context in which they work and to better comprehend current issues and inequalities that impact on communities.

Conclusion

Despite the many challenges to communities in the past 20 years, community work remains an important form of intervention and an important form of practice for sustaining our civil society. The impact of global markets, cutbacks in the public sector, reductions in welfare benefits, low pay, the attempts to turn public services into a market place, and high unemployment rates have made many feel vulnerable and exposed at a time when the small minority of the richest in our society are enjoying substantial increases in their wealth. At the same time the political structures that were created in other times appear unable to respond to the demands for people to express their voice and to be heard and have their needs listened to.

Community work has years of experience, knowledge, and wisdom at being able to provide a realistic tried and tested platform for helping people to articulate the dilemmas they face and a practice to address them. However, many community workers are faced with the impact of increasing managerial control that reflects the employers' lack of trust in and often lack of agreement with their employees' values and judgements. This makes the role of practitioner forums and support groups, as well as engaging with trade unions, an important focus for challenging their employers' negative practices and policies.

The future for community work remains viable and I have great confidence that the choppy seas it faces can be successfully navigated with practitioners, students, academics and citizens generally working together to help create a more just, sustainable and equal society for us and for future generations.

Bibliography

Abel-Smith, B. and Townsend, P. (1965) *The Poor and the Poorest*. London: Bell.

Abrams, P. (1978) *Work, Urbanism and Inequality: UK Society Today*. London: Weidenfeld & Nicolson.

Ackroyd, P. (2001) *London: The Biography*. London: Vintage.

Alcock, C., Daly, G. and Griggs, E. (2008) *Introducing Social Policy*, 2nd edn. Basingstoke: Palgrave Macmillan.

Alinsky, S. (1969) *Reveille for Radicals*. New York: Vintage Books.

Alinsky, S. (1971) *Rules for Radicals: A Pragmatic Reader for Realistic Radicals*. New York: Random House.

Allen, G., Bastiani, J., Martin, I. and Richards, K. (eds) (1987) *Community Education: An Agenda for Educational Reform*. Milton Keynes: Open University Press.

Allen, G. and Martin, I. (eds) (1992) *Education and Community: The Politics of Practice*. London: Cassell.

Allman, P. (1987) Paulo Freire's education: a struggle for meaning, in G. Allen, J. Bastiani, I. Martin and K. Richards (eds), *Community Education: An Agenda for Educational Reform*. Milton Keynes: Open University Press.

Anionwu, E. (1990) Community development approaches to sickle cell anaemia, *Talking Point*, no. 113. Newcastle upon Tyne: Association of Community Workers.

Anthony, P. (1983) *John Ruskin's Labour*. Cambridge: Cambridge University Press.

Arthur, C. (2013) Tech giants may be huge, but nothing matches big data, *The Guardian*, 24 August, p. 6.

Asian Sheltered Residential Accommodation (1981) *Asian Sheltered Residential Accommodation*. London: Asian Sheltered Residential Accommodation.

Bagguley, P. (1991) *From Protest to Acquiescence? Political Movements of the Unemployed*. Basingstoke: Macmillan.

Baldock, P. (1977) Why community action? The historical origins of the radical trend in British community work. *Community Development Journal*, 12(3): 172–81.

Banks, S., Butcher, H., Orton, A. and Robertson, J. (eds) (2013) *Managing Community Practice: Principles, Polices and Programmes*, 2nd edn. Bristol: Policy Press.

Barclay, P. M. (1982) *Social Workers: Their Role and Tasks (The Barclay Report)*. London: Bedford Square Press.

Barker, H. (1986) Recapturing sisterhood: a critical look at 'process' in feminist organising and community work, *Critical Social Policy*, 16, Summer: 80–90.

Barr, A. (1991) *Practising Community Development: Experience in Strathclyde*. London: Community Development Foundation.

Batten, T. R. (1957) *Communities and Their Development*. London: Oxford University Press.

Batten, T. R. (1962) *Training for Community Development: A Critical Study of Method*. London: Oxford University Press.

Batten, T. R. (1965) *The Human Factor in Community Work*. London: Oxford University Press.

Batten, T. R., with the collaboration of Madge Batten (1967) *The Non-directive Approach in Group and Community Work*. London: Oxford University Press.

Batty, E., Beatty, C., Foden, M., Lawless, P., Pearson, S. and Wilson, I. (2010) *The New Deal for Communities Experience: A Final Assessment. The New Deal for Communities Evaluation: Final Report*, Vol. 7. London: Department for Communities and Local Government.

Beck, D. and Purcell, R. (2013) *International Community Organising: Taking Power, Making Change*. Bristol: Policy Press.

Beck, U. (2008) *World at Risk*. Cambridge: Polity.

Bedarida, F. (1990) *A Social History of England 1851–1990* (trans. A. S. Forster and J. Hodgkinson). London: Routledge.

Beilharz, P. (1992) *Labour's Utopias: Bolshevism, Fabianism, Social Democracy*. London: Routledge.

Bell, C. and Newby, H. (1971) *Community Studies*. London: Allen & Unwin.

Benyon, J. and Solomos, J. (1987) *The Roots of Urban Unrest*. Oxford: Pergamon Press.

Bhavnani, K. (1982) Racist acts, *Spare Rib*, 117, April.

Bhavnani, R., Mirza, H. S. and Meeto, V. (2005) *Tackling the Roots of Racism: Lessons for Success*. Bristol: Policy Press.

Biddle, L. and Biddle, W. (1965) *The Community Development Process: The Rediscovery of Local Initiative*. New York: Holt, Rinehart & Winston.

Black, A. (1988) *State, Community and Human Desire*. Brighton: Harvester Wheatsheaf.

Blond, P. (2010) *Red Tory: How Left and Right Have Broken Britain and How We Can Fix It*. London: Faber.

Boal, A. (2008) *Theatre of the Oppressed (Get Political)*. New edn. London: Pluto Press.

Bogdanor, Y. and Skidelsky, R. (1970) *The Age of Affluence, 1951–64*. London: Macmillan.

Bolger, S., Corrigan, P., Docking, J. and Frost, N. (1981) *Towards Socialist Welfare Work*. London: Macmillan.

Briggs, A. and Macartney, A. (1984) *Toynbee Hall: The First Hundred Years*. London: Routledge & Kegan Paul.

Brown, A. (1992) *Groupwork*. London: Heinemann.

Bryant, B. and Bryant, R. (1982) *Change and Conflict: A Study of Community Work in Glasgow*. Aberdeen: Aberdeen University Press.

Bryers, P. (1979) The development of practice theory in community work, *Community Development Journal*, 14(3): 200–9.

Bryson, V. (1993) Feminism, in R. Eatwell and A. Wright (eds) *Contemporary Political Ideology*. London: Pinter.

Buechler, S. M. (1999) *Social Movements in Advanced Capitalism*. Oxford: Oxford University Press.

Burns, D. (1992) *Poll Tax Rebellion*. Stirling and London: AK Press and Attack International.

Butcher, H., Law, I. G., Leach, R. and Mullard, M. (1990) *Local Government and Thatcherism*. London: Routledge.

Butler, D. and Sloman, A. (1976) *British Political Facts, 1900–1975*. London: Macmillan.

Butler, J. (2006) *Gender Trouble: Feminism and the Subversion of Identity*. London: Routledge.

Calder, A. (1971) *The People's War*. London: Panther.

Calouste Gulbenkian Foundation (1968) *Community Work and Social Change*. London: Longman.

Cannan, C. (2000) The environmental crisis, greens and community development, *Community Development Journal*, 35(4): 365–76.

Carroll, J. M. (2007) *A Concise History of Hong Kong*. Hong Kong: Hong Kong University Press.

Castells, M. (1975) Advanced capitalism, collective consumption and urban contradictions, in L. Lindberg, R. Alford, C. Crouch, and C. Offe (eds) *Stress and Contradictions in Modern Capitalism*. London: Lexington Books.

Castells, M. (1977) *The Urban Question*. London: Edward Arnold.

Castells, M. (2000a) *The Rise of the Network Society: The Information Age: Economy, Society and Culture*, Vol. I. Oxford: Blackwell.

Castells, M. (2000b) *The Rise of the Network Society: The Information Age: Economy, Society and Culture*, Vol. II. Oxford: Blackwell.

Castells, M. (2004) *The Rise of the Network Society: The Information Society: Economy, Society and Culture*, Vol. II. Oxford: Blackwell.

Castells, M. (2012) *Networks of Outrage and Hope: Social Movements in the Internet Age*. Cambridge: Polity Press.

CDF (2007) *The Community Development Challenge*. London: Community Development Foundation.

CDP (1977) *Gilding the Ghetto: The State and the Poverty Experiments*. London: Community Development Project Inter-project Editorial Team.

Chambers, D. (2006) *New Social Ties: Contemporary Connections in a Fragmented Society*. Basingstoke: Palgrave.

Chanan, G. (2003) *Searching for Solid Foundations: Community Involvement and Urban Policy*. London: Office of the Deputy Prime Minister.

Cheetham, J. (1988) Ethnic associations in Britain, in S. Jenkins (ed.) *Ethnic Associations and the Welfare State*. New York: Columbia University Press.

Clark, D. (1983) The concept of community education, *Journal of Community Education*, 2(3): 34–41.

Coates, K. and Silburn, R. (1970) *Poverty: The Forgotten Englishmen*. Harmondsworth: Penguin.

Cochrane, A. (1993) *Whatever Happened to Local Government?* Buckingham: Open University Press.

Cockburn, C. (1977) *The Local State*. London: Pluto Press.

Cole, G. D. H. (1918) *Self Government in Industry*. London: Bell.

Cole, G. D. H. (1920) *Guild Socialism Re-stated*. London: Parsons.

Cole, M. I. (ed.) (1956) *Beatrice Webb's Diaries, 1924–1932*. London: Fabian Society.

Collins, P. H. (2000) *Black Feminist Thought: Knowledge, Consciousness and the Politics of Empowerment*. New York: Routledge.

Community Matters (2011) Demand up and income down at Britain's community centres, 17 October, Press release. London: Community Matters.

Cooper, N., Purcell, S. and Jackson, R. (2014) *Below the Breadline: The Relentless Rise of Food Poverty in Britain*. Oxford: Church Action on Poverty, The Tressell Trust and Oxfam.

Corkey, D. and Craig, G. (1978) Community Work or Class Politics?' in P. Curno, (ed.), *Political Issues and Community Work*. London: Routledge & Kegan Paul.

Cornwell, J. (1984) *Hard Earned Lives*. London: Tavistock.

Council of Europe (2006) *Campaign to Combat Violence against Women, Including Domestic Violence*. Fact sheet, available at: www.coe.int/t/dg2/equality/domesticviolencecampaign/fact_sheet_en.asp

Coutts, K. and Godley, W. (1989) The British economy under Mrs Thatcher, *Political Quarterly*, Summer, 60(2): 137–51.

Cowley, J., Kaye, A., Mayo, M. and Thompson, M. (1977) *Community or Class Struggle*. London: Stage 1.

Craig, G. (1989) Community work and the state, *Community Development Journal*, 24(1): 3–18.

Craig, G., Derricourt, N. and Loney, M. (eds) (1982) *Community Work and the State: Towards a Radical Practice: Community Work Eight*. London: Routledge & Kegan Paul in association with the Association of Community Workers.

Craig, G., Mayo, M., Popple, K., Shaw, M. and Taylor, M. (eds) (2011) *The Community Development Reader: History, Themes and Issues*. Bristol: Policy Press.

Craig, G., Mayo, M. and Sharman, N. (1979) *Jobs and Community Action: Community Work Five*. London: Routledge & Kegan Paul in association with the Association of Community Workers.

Craig, G., Popple, K. and Shaw, M. (eds) (2008) *Community Development in Theory and Practice: An International Reader*. Nottingham: Spokesman Books.

Cumella, M. (1984) Community work and unemployment: the aftermath of the 'slimline' of the steel industry in Newport, South Wales, *COMM*, 22, August. Marcinelle, Belgium: Inter-University European Institute of Social Welfare.

Curno, A., Lamming, A., Leach, L., Stiles, J., Ward, V. and Ziff, T. (1982) *Women in Collective Action*. Newcastle upon Tyne: Association of Community Workers.

Curno, P. (ed.) (1978) *Political Issues and Community Work: Community Work Four*. London: Routledge & Kegan Paul.

Darner, S. (1980) State, class and housing: Glasgow 1875–1919, in J. Melling (ed.) *Housing, Social Policy and the State*. London: Croom Helm.

Dearlove, J. (1974) The control of change and the regulations of community action, in D. Jones and M. Mayo (eds) *Community Work One*. London: Routledge & Kegan Paul.

Debord, G. (1997) Introduction to a critique of urban geography, in G. Debord (ed.) *Theory of the Derive*. New York: Atlantic Books.

Demuth, C. (1977) *Government Initiatives on Urban Deprivation*. London: Runnymede Trust.

Denborough, D. (2008) *Collective Narrative Practice: Responding to Individuals, Groups and Communities Who Have Experienced Trauma*. Adelaide: Dulwich Centre Publications.

DES (1967) *Children and Their Primary Schools*. Report to the Central Advisory Council for Education, No. 1 (the Plowden Report). London: HMSO.

DES (1969) *Youth and Community Work in the 1970s. Proposals by the Youth Service Development Council* (the Fairbairn-Milson Report). London: HMSO.

DHSS (1989) *Caring for People: Community Care in the Next Decade and Beyond*. London: HMSO.

Dixon, G., Johnson, C., Leigh, S. and Turnbull, N. (1982) Feminist perspectives and practice, in G. Craig, N. Derricourt, and M. Loney (eds) *Community Work and the State: Towards a Radical Practice: Community Work Eight*. London: Routledge & Kegan Paul.

Dobson, A. and Bell, D. (eds) (2006) *Environmental Citizenship*. Cambridge, MA: MIT Press.

Dominelli, L. (2002) *Feminist Social Work Theory and Practice*. Basingstoke: Macmillan.

Dominelli, L. (2006) *Women and Community Action*, revised 2nd edn. Bristol: Policy Press.

Edwards, J. and Batley, R. (1978) *The Politics of Positive Discrimination*. London: Tavistock.

Edwards, M. and Gaventa, J. (2001) *Global Citizen Action*. London: Earthscan.

Elliott, L. (2012) A new world order – but not in the way Brown meant, *The Guardian*. 11 June, p. 17.

Ellison, D. (1988) Community work and E.T., *Talking Point*, no. 98, November. Newcastle upon Tyne: Association of Community Workers.

Emejulu, A. (2011) Re-theorizing feminist community development: towards a radical democratic citizenship, *Community Development Journal*, 46(3): 378–90.

Emejulu, A. and Shaw, M. (eds) (2010) *Community Empowerment Critical Perspectives from Scotland. The Glasgow Papers*. Edinburgh: Community Development Journal.

Engels, F. (1844) *The Condition of the English Working Class*. London: Paladin.

Etzioni, A. (1995) *The Spirit of Community*. London: Fontana.

Fairbairn, A. (1979) *The Leicestershire Community Colleges and Centres*. Nottingham: Nottingham University/National Institute for Adult Education.

FCDL (2009) *National Occupational Standards for Community Development*. Sheffield: Federation of Community Development Learning.

Finn, D. (1987) *Training without Jobs: New Deals and Broken Promises*. London: Macmillan.

Flynn, R. and Craig, G. (2012) Policy, politics and practice: a historical review and its relevance to current debates, in G. Craig, K. Atkin, S. Chattoo, and R. Flynn *Understanding 'Race' and Ethnicity: Theory, History, Policy, Practice*. Bristol: Policy Press.

Foot, P. (1969) *The Rise of Enoch Powell: An Examination of Enoch Powell's Attitude to Immigration and Race*. Harmondsworth: Penguin.

Fortune (2006) Global 500, 4 July.

Foucault, M. (1967) *Madness and Civilisation: A History of Insanity*. London: Tavistock.

Foucault, M. (1977) *Discipline and Punishment: The Birth of the Prison*. Harmondsworth: Allen Lane.

Foucault, M. (1980) *Power/Knowledge: Selected Interviews and Other Writings, 1972–1977*. C. Gordon (ed.). Brighton: Harvester Press.

Francis, D., Henderson, P. and Thomas, D. N. (1984) *A Survey of Community Workers in the United Kingdom*. London: National Institute for Social Work.

Frankenberg, R. (1969) *Communities in Britain: Social Life in Town and Country*. Harmondsworth: Penguin Books.

Fraser, D. (1984) *The Evolution of the British Welfare State*, 2nd edn. London: Macmillan.

Fraser, J. (1987) Community: the private and the individual, *Journal of Sociological Review*, 35(4): 795–818.

Fraser, N. (1989) *Unruly Practices: Power, Discourse and Gender in Contemporary Social Theory*. Cambridge: Polity.

Freeman, J. (1984) *The Tyranny of Structurelessness*. London: Dark Star and Rebel Press.

Freire, P. (1970) *Cultural Action for Freedom*. Harmondsworth: Penguin.

Freire, P. (1972) *Pedagogy of the Oppressed*. Harmondsworth: Penguin.

Freire, P. (1976) *Education: The Practice of Freedom*. London: Writers and Readers Publishing Cooperative.

Freire, P. (1985) *The Politics of Education: Culture, Power and Liberation*. London: Macmillan.

Fromm, E. (1969) *Escape from Freedom*. New York: Avon Books.

Gallacher, J., Ohri, A. and Roberts, L. (1983) Unemployment and community action, *Community Development Journal*, 18(1): 2–9.

Gamble, A. (1987) The weakening of social democracy, in M. Loney, R. Bocock, J. Clarke, A. Cochrane, P. Graham and M. Wilson (eds) *The State or the Market: Politics and Welfare in Contemporary Britain*. London: Sage/Open University Press.

Geraghty, C. (1991) *Women and Soap Operas*. Cambridge: Polity.

Giddens, A. (1998) *The Third Way: The Renewal of Social Democracy*. Cambridge: Polity.

Giddens, A. and Sutton, P. W. (2013) *Sociology*, 7th edn. Cambridge: Polity.

Gilchrist, A. (1992) The revolution of everyday life revisited: towards an anti-discriminatory praxis for community work, *Social Action*, 1(1): 22–8.

Gilchrist, A. and Taylor, M. (2011) *The Short Guide to Community Development*. Bristol: Policy Press.

Gillis, S., Howie, G. and Mumford, R. (2007) *Third Wave Feminism: A Critical Exploration*, 2nd edn. Basingstoke: Palgrave Macmillan.

Gilroy, P. (1993) *Small Acts: Thoughts on the Politics of Black Cultures*. London: Serpent's Tail.

Glen, A., Henderson, P., Humm, J., Meszaros, H. with Gaffney, M. (2004) *Survey of Community Development Workers in the UK*. Sheffield: Community Development Exchange.

Goetschius, G. (1975) Some difficulties in introducing a community work option into social work training, in D. Jones and M. Mayo (eds), *Community Work Two*. London: Routledge & Kegan Paul.

Goffman, E. (1961) *Asylums*. New York: Doubleday.

Golding, P. and Sills, A. (1983) Community against itself: social communication in the urban community, *COMM*, 20, December: 177–94. Marcinelle, Belgium: Inter-University European Institute of Social Welfare.

Goodson, L. and Phillimore, J. (eds) (2012) *Community Research for Participation: From Theory to Method*. Bristol: Policy Press.

Goodwin, M. and Duncan, S. (1986) The local state and local economic policy: political mobilisation or economic regeneration, *Capital and Class*, 27, Winter: 14–36.

Gough, I. (1979) *The Political Economy of the Welfare State*. London: Macmillan.

Gouldbourne, H. (1998) *Race Relations in Britain since 1945*. London: Macmillan Press.

Graef, R. (1989) *Talking Blues*. London: Collins.

Gramsci, A. (1971) *Selections from the Prison Notebooks* (ed. and trans. Q. Hoare and G. Nowell Smith). London: Lawrence and Wishart.

Gramsci, A. (1975) *Letters from Prison* (selected and trans. J. Lawner). London: Jonathan Cape.

Gramsci, A. (1977) *Selections from Political Writings 1910–1920* (ed. Q. Hoare). London: Lawrence and Wishart.

Gramsci, A. (1978) *Selections from Political Writings 1921–1926* (ed. Q. Hoare). London: Lawrence and Wishart.

Grant, D. (1989) *Learning Relations*. London: Routledge.

Gray, M. (2010) Social development and the status quo: professionalization and the third way cooptation, *International Journal of Social Welfare*, 19(4): 463–70.

Gray, M. and Boddy, J. (2010) Making sense of the waves: wipeout or still riding high? *Affilia*, 25(4): 368–89.

Green, J. (1992) The community project revisited, in P. Carter, T. Jeffs, and M.K. Smith (eds) *Changing Social Work and Welfare*. Buckingham: Open University Press.

Green, J. and Chapman, A. (1990) The lessons of the CDP for community development today, paper delivered at the OU/HEC Winter School, 'Roots and Branches: Community Development and Health'.

Hadley, R., Cooper, M., Dale, P. and Stacey, G. (1987) *A Community Social Worker's Handbook*. London: Tavistock.

Hall, S. (1988) *The Hard Road to Renewal: Thatcherism and the Crisis of the Left*. London: Verso.

Hall, S. (2006) New ethnicities, in B. Ashcroft, G. Griffiths and H. Tiffin (eds) *The Post-Colonial Studies Reader*, 2nd edn. London: Routledge.

Halpern, M. (1963) *The Politics of Social Change in the Middle East and North Africa*. Princeton, NJ: Princeton University Press.

Halsey, A. H. (ed.) (1972) *Educational Priority*. London: HMSO.

Hanmer, J. and Rose, H. (1980) Making sense of theory, in P. Henderson, D. Jones and D. N. Thomas (eds) *The Boundaries of Change in Community Work*. London: Allen & Unwin.

Hanmer, J. and Statham, D. (1988) *Women and Social Work: Towards a Woman-Centred Practice*. Basingstoke: Macmillan.

Hannington, W. (1967) *Never on Our Knees*. London: Lawrence & Wishart.

Hannington, W. (1977) *Unemployed Struggles, 1919–1936.* London: Lawrence & Wishart.

Hanson, D. (1972) Community centres and their functions as educational institutions and agencies for social control, *Durham Review*, 28.

Harris, J. (1977) *William Beveridge: A Biography.* Oxford: Clarendon Press.

Harris, J. (1981) Social policy making in Britain during the Second World War, in W. Mommsen (ed.), *The Emergence of the Welfare State in Britain and Germany.* London: Croom Helm.

Harris, L. (1988) The UK economy at a crossroads, in J. Allen and D. Massey (eds) *The Economy in Question.* London: Sage.

Harris, V. (2009) *Community Work Skills Manual.* Sheffield: Federation of Community Development Learning.

Hazekamp, J. L. and Popple, K. (eds) (1997) *Racism in Europe: A Challenge for Youth Policy and Youth Work.* London: UCL Press.

Held, D., McGrew, A., Goldblatt, D. and Perraton, J. (1999) *Global Transformation: Politics, Economics and Culture.* Cambridge: Polity.

Henderson, P. (1983) The contribution of the CDP to the development of community work, in D. N. Thomas (ed.) *Community Work in the Eighties.* London: National Institute of Social Work.

Henderson, P. and Thomas, D. (2013) *Skills in Neighbourhood Work*, 4th edn. London: Routledge.

Henderson, P. and Vercseg, I. (2010) *Community Development and Civil Society: Making Connections in the European Context.* Bristol: Policy Press.

Henderson, P., Wright, A. and Wyncoll, K. (eds) (1982) *Successes and Struggles on Council Estates: Tenant Action and Community Work.* London: Association of Community Workers.

Heraud, B. (1975) The new towns: a philosophy of community,' in P. Leonard (ed.) *The Sociology of Community Action.* Sociological Review Monograph 21. Keele: University of Keele.

Hill, G. (1987) Community work and the MSC, *Talking Point*, no. 85, July. Newcastle upon Tyne: Association of Community Workers.

Hills, J., Brewer, M., Jenkins, S. P., Lister, R., Lupton, R., Machin, S., Mills, C., Modood, T., Rees, T. and Riddell, S. (2010) *An Anatomy of Economic Inequality in the UK: Report of the National Equality Panel.* London: Government Equalities Office.

HMSO (1954) *Social Development in the British Colonial Territories.* Report of the Ashbridge Conference on Social Development (Colonial Office), 3–12 August. London: HMSO.

HMSO (1968) *Report of the Committee on Local Authority and Applied Personal Social Services*, Cmnd. 3703 (the Seebohm Report). London: HMSO.

HMSO (1969) *People and Planning* (the Skeffington Report). London: HMSO.

HMSO (1981) *The Brixton Disorders 10–12 April 1981: Report of an Inquiry by the Rt. Hon. the Lord Scarman, QBE*, Cmnd. 8427 (the Scarman Report). London: HMSO.

Hobsbawm, E. J. (1968) Poverty, in D. L. Sills (ed.) *New International Encyclopaedia of the Social Sciences*, vol. 12. London: Macmillan.

Home Office (1960) *Children and Young Persons* (the Ingleby Report). London: HMSO.

hooks, b. (1981) *Ain't I a Woman?: Black Women and Feminism*. Boston, MA: South End Press.

hooks, b. (1993) bell hooks speaking about Paulo Freire: the man, his work, in P. McLaren and P. Leonard (eds), *Paulo Freire: A Critical Encounter*. London: Routledge.

hooks, b. (1994) *Teaching to Transgress: Education as the Practice of Freedom*. New York: Routledge.

hooks, b. (1997) *Bone Black: Memories of Girlhood*. London: Women's Press.

Hopkins, R. (2011) *The Transition Companion: Making your Community More Resilient in Uncertain Times*. Totnes: Green Books.

Howe, D. (1987) *An Introduction to Social Work Theory*. Aldershot: Gower.

Hutton, W. (1993) Slouching towards a recovery, *Guardian*, 18 March.

IACD (2013) *IACD Annual Review*. Falkland: International Association for Community Development.

Iliffe, S. (1985) The politics of health care: the NHS under Thatcher, *Critical Social Policy*, 14: 57–72.

Jacobs, S. and Popple, K. (eds) (1994) Community Work in the 1990s. Nottiingham: Spokesman.

Jeffs, A. J. (1979) *Young People and the Youth Service*. London: Routledge & Kegan Paul.

Jenkins, S. (2004) *Big Bang Localism: A Rescue Plan for British Democracy*. London: Policy Exchange and Localis.

Johnson, C. (1991) *The Economy under Mrs Thatcher 1979–1990*. London: Penguin Books.

Jones, D. (1977) Community work in the United Kingdom, in H. Specht and A. Vickery (eds) *Integrating Social Work Methods*. London: Allen & Unwin.

Jones, D. (1983) Community of interest: a reprise, in D. N. Thomas (ed.) *Community Work in the Eighties*. London: National Institute of Social Work.

Jones, D. and Mayo, M. (eds) (1975) *Community Work Two*. London: Routledge & Kegan Paul.

Jones, L. (1986) The Community Programme Scheme, *Talking Point*, no. 77, October. Newcastle upon Tyne: Association of Community Workers.

Jordan, B. and Drakeford, M. (2012) *Social Work and Social Policy under Austerity*. Basingstoke: Palgrave Macmillan.

Joseph, K. (1972) The next ten years, *New Society*, 5 October.

Judd, D. (1996) *Empire: The British Imperial Experience from 1765 to the Present*. London: HarperCollins.

Kalka, I. (1991) The politics of the 'community' among Gujarati Hindus in London, *New Community*, 17(3): 377–85.

Kane, D., Bass, P., Heywood, J., Jochum, V., James, D. and Lloyd, G. (2014) *UK Civil Society Almanac*. London: National Council for Voluntary Organisations.

Kettle, M. (1988) Years of revolution, in *68/88*. London: Channel 4 Television.

Kraut, R., Bryin, M. and Kielser, S. (eds) (2006) *Computers, Phones and the Internet: Domesticating Internet Technology*. Buckingham: Open University Press.

Krolloke, C. and Sorensen, A.S. (2006) *Gender Communication Theories and Analyses: From Silence to Performance*. London: Sage.

Kuenstler, P. (1961) *Community Organisations in Great Britain*. London: Faber.

Kuper, B. (1985) The supply of training, *Youth and Policy*, 13, Summer: 15–18.

Kwo, E. M. (1984) Community education and community development in Cameroon: the British colonial experience, 1922–1961, *Community Development Journal*, 19(4): 204–13.

Lamoureux, H., Mayer, R. and Panet-Raymond, J. (1989) *Community Action*. Quebec: Black Rose Books.

Langan, M. (1990) Community care in the 1990s: the community care White Paper: 'Caring for People', *Critical Social Policy*, 29, Autumn: 58–70.

Lansley, S. (2011) *The Cost of Inequality: Three Decades of the Super-Rich and the Economy*. London: Gibson Square.

Lapping, A. (ed.) (1970) *Community Action* (Fabian Tract 400). London: Fabian Society.

Laurence, S. and Hall, P. (1981) British policy responses, in P. Hall (ed.) *The Inner City in Context: The Final Report of the Social Science Research Council Inner Cities Working Party*. Aldershot: Gower.

Law, I. (2010) *Racism and Ethnicity: Global Debates, Dilemmas, Directions*. Harlow: Pearson.

Leaper, R. A. B. (1971) *Community Work*. London: National Council of Social Service.

Ledwith, M. (2011) *Community Development: A Critical Approach*, 2nd edn. Bristol: Policy Press.

Ledwith, M. and Spingett, J. (2010) *Participatory Practice: Community-Based Action for Transformative Change*. Bristol: Policy Press.

Lees, R. and Mayo, M. (1984) *Community Action for Change*. London: Routledge & Kegan Paul.

Leonard, P. (ed.) (1975) *The Sociology of Community Action*, Sociological Review Monograph 21. Keele: University of Keele.

Lister, R. (2001) New Labour: a study in ambiguity from a position of ambivalence, *Critical Social Policy*, 21(69): 425–48.

Lomax, E. (2005) *The Railway Man*. London: Vintage.

London Edinburgh Weekend Return Group (1980) *In and Against the State*. London: Pluto Press.

Loney, M. (1983) *Community against Government: The British Community Development Project 1968–78*. London: Heinemann Educational Books.

Loudon, J. B. (1961) Kinship and crisis in South Wales, *British Journal of Sociology*, XII(4): 333–40.

Lovell, G. (2009) T.R. Batten's life and work, in R. Gilchrist, T. Jeffs, T. Spence and J. Walker (eds) *Essays in the History of Youth and Community Work: Discovering the Past*. Lyme Regis: Russell House Publishing.

Lovett, T. (1975) *Adult Education, Community Development and the Working Class*. London: Ward Lock.

Lovett, T., Clarke, C. and Kilmurray, A. (1983) *Adult Education and Community Action*. London: Croom Helm.

Lukes, S. (2005) *Power: A Radical View*, 2nd edn. Basingstoke: Palgrave Macmillan.

Macpherson, S. W. (1999) *The Stephen Lawrence Inquiry*. Cm 4262-I. London: HMSO.

Marr, A. (2007) *A History of Modern Britain*. London: Macmillan.

Marsden, D. and Oakley, P. (1982) Radical community development in the Third World, in G. Craig, N. Derricourt and M. Loney (eds) *Community Work and the State: Community Work Eight*. London: Routledge & Kegan Paul.

Martin, I. (1987) Community education: towards a theoretical analysis, in G. Allen, J. Bastiani, I. Martin and K. Richards (eds) *Community Education: An Agenda for Educational Reform*. Milton Keynes: Open University Press.

Marwick, A. (2000) *A History of the Modern British Isles, 1914–1999*. Oxford: Blackwell.

Mason, P. (2012) *Why It's Kicking Off Everywhere: The New Global Revolutions*. London: Verso.

Mayo, M. (1975) The history and early development of CDP, in R. Lees and G. Smith (eds) *Action Research in Community Development*. London: Routledge & Kegan Paul.

Mayo, M. (ed.) (1977) *Women in the Community: Community Work Three*. London: Routledge & Kegan Paul.

Mayo, M. (1980) Beyond CDP: reaction and community action, in R. Bailey and M. Brake (eds) *Radical Social Work and Practice*. London: Edward Arnold.

Mayo, M. (1982) Community Action Programmes in the early eighties: what future?, *Critical Social Policy*, 1(3): 5–18.

Mayo, M. (2008) Community development, contestations, continuities and change, in G. Craig, K. Popple and M. Shaw (eds) *Community Development in Theory and Practice: An International Reader*. Nottingham: Spokesman Books.

Mayo, M. and Jones, D. (eds) (1974) *Community Work One*. London: Routledge & Kegan Paul.

Mayo, M., Mendiwelso-Bendek, Z. and Packham, C. (eds) (2013) *Community Research for Community Development*. Basingstoke: Palgrave Macmillan.

Mayo, M. and Robertson, J. (2013) The historical and policy context: setting the scene for current debates, in S. Banks, H. Butcher, A. Orton and J. Robertson (eds) *Managing Community Practice: Principles, Polices and Programmes*, 2nd edn. Bristol: Policy Press.

McCloy, R. (2013) The Cambridgeshire Village College: origin and mutation, a perspective, in R. Gilchrist, T. Jeffs, J. Spence, N. Stanton, A. Cowell, J. Walker and T. Wylie (eds) *Reappraisals: Essays in the History of Youth and Community Work*. Lyme Regis: Russell House.

McConnell, C. (2002) *Community Learning and Development: The Making of an Empowering Profession*. Edinburgh: Community Learning Scotland/PAULO.

McKay, D. and Cox, A. (1979) *The Politics of Urban Change*. London: Croom Helm.

McMichael, P., Lynch, B. and Wright, D. (1990) *Building Bridges into Work: The Role of the Community Worker*. Harlow: Longman.

Meier, P. (1978) *William Morris: The Marxist Dreamer* (trans. F. Gubb). Brighton: Harvester.

Melling, J. (1980) Clydeside housing and the evolution of state rent control, in J. Melling (ed.) *Housing, Social Policy and the State*. London: Croom Helm.

Midwinter, E. (1972) *Priority Education*. Harmondsworth: Penguin.

Midwinter, E. (1975) *Education and the Community*. London: George Allen & Unwin.

Millet, K. (1969) *Sexual Politics*. London: Abacus.

Mills, R. (1983) Trusts and Foundations as innovative bodies, in D. N. Thomas (ed.) *Community Work in the Eighties*. London: National Institute for Social Work.

Mirowski, P. (2013) *Never Let a Serious Crisis Go to Waste: How Neoliberalism Survived the Financial Meltdown*. London: Verso.

Monbiot, G. (2014) The rich want us to believe their wealth is good for us all, *The Guardian*. 30 July.

Mondros, J. B. and Wilson, S. M. (1994) *Organizing for Power and Empowerment*. New York: Columbia University Press.

Morris, H. (1925) *The Village College: Being a Memorandum on the Provision of Educational and Social Facilities for the Countryside, with Special Reference to Cambridgeshire*. Cambridge: Cambridge University Press.

Morris, J., Cobbing, P. and Leach, K. with Conaty (finance report) (2013) *Mainstreaming Community Economic Development: Localise West Midlands*. Birmingham: Localise West Midlands.

Mowatt, C. L. (1961) *The Charity Organisation Society, 1869–1913: Its Ideas and Work*. London: Methuen.

Mukhopadhyay, A. R. (2007) Radical Islam in Europe: misperceptions and misconception, in T. Abbas (ed.) *Islamic Political Radicalism: A European Perspective*. Edinburgh: Edinburgh University Press.

Ng, R. (1988) *The Politics of Community Services: Immigrant Women, Class and the State*. Toronto: Garamond Press.

Ohri, A., Manning, B. and Curno, P. (eds) (1982) *Community Work and Racism: Community Work Seven*. London: Routledge & Kegan Paul in association with the Association of Community Workers.

Ohri, A. and Roberts, L. (1981) Can community workers do anything about unemployment?, *Talking Point*, no. 28. London: Association of Community Workers.

O'Malley, J. (1977) *Politics of Community Action*. London: Russell.

ONS (2012) *Ethnicity and National Identity in England and Wales 2011*. London: Office for National Statistics.

Orwell, G. (2013) *Nineteen Eighty-Four*. London: Penguin Classics.

Oxfam (2014a) *Working for the Few: Political Capture and Economic Inequality*. Oxfam Briefing Paper 178. Oxford: Oxfam GB.

Oxfam (2014b) *A Tale of Two Britains*. Oxfam Media Briefing Paper. Oxford: Oxfam GB.

Pahl, R. E. (1966) The rural-urban continuum, *Sociologia Ruralis*, 6: 299–329.

Parekh, B. (2000) *Rethinking Multiculturalism*. Cambridge, MA: Harvard University Press.

Parker, R.A. (1981) Tending and social policy, in E. M. Goldberg and S. Hatch (eds), *A New Look at the Personal Social Services*. London: Policy Studies Institute.

Parry, N. and Parry, J. (1979) Social work, professionalism and the state, in N. Parry, M. Rustin and C. Satyamurti (eds) *Social Work, Welfare and the State*. London: Edward Arnold.

Payne, M. (2005) *The Origins of Social Work: Continuity and Change*. Basingstoke: Palgrave Macmillan.

Pearson, G. (1983) *Hooligan: A History of Respectable Fears*. London: Macmillan.

Peatfield, P. (1992) *The Only Step in the Line: The Lone Manager in the Small Voluntary Organisation*. London: Centre for Voluntary Organisations.

Pitchford, M. with Henderson, P. (2008) *Making Spaces for Community Development*. Bristol: Policy Press in association with the Community Development Foundation.

Piven, F. and Cloward, R. (1977) *Poor People's Movement Why They Succeed, How They Fail*. New York: Vintage Books.

Popple, K. (1994) Towards a progressive community work praxis, in S. Jacobs and K. Popple (eds) *Community Work in the 1990's*. Nottingham: Spokesman.

Popple, K. (2002) *Making Sense of Community*. On Learning, Teaching and Higher Education working papers. Vol. 1, Working Paper 14. Southampton: Southampton Institute.

Popple, K. (2003) The *Community Development Journal*: a history, in R. Gilchrist, T. Jeffs, and J. Spence (eds) *Architects of Change: Studies in the History of Community and Youth Work*. Leicester: National Youth Agency.

Popple, K. (2008) The first forty years of the *Community Development Journal*, *Community Development Journal*, 43(1): 6–23.

Popple, K. (2009) The counter-cultural revolution and the OZ School Kids issue: the establishment versus the underground press, in R. Gilchrist, T, Jeffs, J. Spence and J. Walker (eds) *Essays in the History of Youth and Community Work: Discovering the Past*. Lyme Regis: Russell House Publishing.

Popple, K. (2011) Rise and fall of the National Community Development Projects, 1968–1978: lessons to learn? in R. Gilchrist, T. Hodgson, T. Jeffs, J. Spence,

N. Stanton and J. Walker (eds) *Reflecting on the Past: Essays in the History of Youth and Community Work.* Lyme Regis: Russell House Publishing.

Popple, K. (2012) Community practice, in M. Gray, J. Midgley and S. A. Webb (eds) *The SAGE Handbook of Social Work.* London: SAGE.

Popple, K. (2013) Reconsidering the 1950s and 1960s: the emergence and establishment of community development in the UK, in R. Gilchrist, T. Jeffs, J. Spence, N. Stanton, A. Cowell, J. Walker and T. Wylie (eds) *Reappraisals: Essays in the History of Youth and Community Work.* Lyme Regis: Russell House.

Powell, E. (1968) Text of speech delivered in Birmingham, 20 April 1968, *Race*, X(1): 80–104.

Powell, F. and Geoghegan, M. (2004) *The Politics of Community Development.* Dublin: A. & A. Farmar.

Procter, J. (2004) *Stuart Hall.* London: Routledge.

Purcell, R. (1982) Community action and real work, *Talking Point*, No. 32. London: Association of Community Workers.

Putman, R. (2000) *Bowling Alone: The Collapse and Revival of American Community.* New York: Simon & Schuster.

Radford, J. (1970) From King Hill to the Squatting Association, in A. Lapping (ed.) *Community Action* (Fabian Tract 400). London: Fabian Society.

Ree, H. (1973) *Educator Extraordinary: The Life and Achievements of Henry Morris.* London: Longman.

Ree, H. (1985) *The Henry Morris Collection.* Cambridge: Cambridge University Press.

Reid, L., Hunter, C. and Sutton, P. (2009) Writing it down: suggestions for a new approach towards understanding pro-environmental behavior, *International Journal of Sustainable Development and World Ecology*, 16 (6): 369–73.

Rimmer, J. (1980) *Troubles Shared: The Story of a Settlement, 1899–1979.* Birmingham: Phlogiston.

Roberts, J. (2006) Making a place for Muslim youth work in British youth work, *Youth and Policy*, 92, Summer.

Robertson, C. (1991) Moral trust comes before skills and information technology, *Talking Point*, no. 122. Newcastle upon Tyne: Association of Community Workers.

Robertson, D. (1985) *The Penguin Dictionary of Politics.* London: Penguin.

Rogers, V. (1994) Feminist work and community education, in S. Jacobs and K. Popple (eds) *Community Work in the 1990s.* Nottingham: Spokesman.

Roof (1986) The penny drops at Coin Street, *Roof*, March/April: 6–7.

Rosenberg, J.D. (1961) *The Darkening Glass.* New York: Columbia University Press.

Ross, M. (1955) *Community Organisation: Theory, Principles and Practice.* New York: Harper and Row.

Rothman, J. (1970) Three models of community organisation practice, in F. Cox, J. Erlich, J. Rothman and J. Tropman (eds), *Strategies of Community Organisation.* Itaska, IL: Peacock Publishing.

Rowbotham, S. (1977) *Hidden from History*. London: Pluto Press.

Rowbotham, S. (1979) Women: how far have we come?, *Hackney People's Press*, November; reprinted in Rowbotham, S. (1983), *Dreams and Dilemmas*. London: Virago.

Rowbotham, S. (1989) *The Past Is Before Us: Feminism in Action since the 1960s*. London: Penguin.

Rowbotham, S. (1992) *Women in Movement: Feminism and Social Action*. London: Routledge.

Rutter, J., Cooley, L., Reynolds, S. and Sheldon, R. (2007) *From Refugee to Citizen: 'Standing on My Own Two Feet'*. London: Refugee Support.

Salmon, H. (1984) *Unemployment: The Two Nations*. London: Association of Community Workers.

Scase, R. (1992) *Class*. Buckingham: Open University Press.

Seabrook, J. (1984) *The Idea of Neighbourhood: What Local Politics Should Be About*. London: Pluto Press.

Selbourne, D. (2014) The defence of reason, *New Statesman*, 18–24 July.

Sen, A. (2001) *Development as Freedom*. Oxford: Oxford University Press.

Sen, A. (2007) *Identity and Violence: The Illusion of Destiny*. London: Penguin.

Sender, H., Carlisle, B., Hatamian, A. and Bowles, M. (2010) *Report on Survey of Community Development Practitioners and Managers*. London: Community Development Foundation.

Shaw, M. (2004) *Community Work: Policy, Politics and Practice*. Hull and Edinburgh: Universities of Hull and Edinburgh.

Sheridan, L. P. (2006) Islamophobia pre-and post-September 11th 2001, *Journal of Interpersonal Violence*, 21: 317–36.

Shukra, K. (2007) The changing terrain of multi-culture: from anti-oppressive practice to community cohesion, *Concept*, 17(3): 3–17.

Silburn, R. (1971) The potential and limitations of community action, in D. Bull (ed.) *Family Poverty*. London: Duckworth & Co.

Simon, R. (1982) *Gramsci's Political Thought*. London: Lawrence & Wishart.

Sinclair, I. (2003) *Lights out for a Territory*. Harmondsworth: Penguin.

Sked, A. and Cook, C. (1984) *Post-War Britain: A Political History*, 2nd edn. London: Penguin.

Skills-Third Sector (2013) *The UK Voluntary Sector Workforce Almanac*. London: Skills-Third Sector.

Skinner, S. (1997) *Building Community Strengths: A Resource Book on Capacity Building*. London: Community Development Foundation.

Smith, I. (1980) Community work and 'qualifications', *Talking Point*, no. 19. London: Association of Community Workers.

Smith, I. (1989) Community work in recession: a practioner's perspective, in M. Langan and P. Lee (eds) *Radical Social Work Today*. London: Unwin Hyman.

Smith, L. and Jones, D. (eds) (1981) *Deprivation, Participation and Communication Action. Community Work Six*. London: Routledge & Kegan Paul.

Smith, M. (1979) Concepts of community work: a British view, in D. A. Chekki (ed.) *Community Development: Theory and Method of Manned Change*. New Delhi: Vika Publishing House.

Smith, M. J. (1998) *Ecologism: Towards Ecological Citizenship*. Buckingham: Open University Press.

Smith, M. J. and Pangsapa, P. (2008) *Environment and Citizenship: Integrating Justice, Responsibility and Civic Engagement*. London: Zed Books.

Smithies, J. and Webster, G. (1987) Feminist organising and community work: a response to Hilary Barker, 'Recapturing Sisterhood', *Critical Social Policy*, 20: 83–5.

Somerville, P. (2011) *Understanding Community: Politics, Policy and Practice*. Bristol: Policy Press.

Sondhi, R. (1982) The Asian Resource Centre, in J. Cheetham (ed.) *Ethnicity and Social Work*. Oxford: Oxford University Press.

Soni, S. (2011) *Working with Diversity in Youth and Community Work*. Exeter: Learning Matters.

Spence, J. (1985) Unemployment, youth and national community service, *Youth and Policy*, 13, Summer: 6–11.

Stacey, M. (1969) The myth of community studies, *British Journal of Sociology*, 20: 134–47.

Stanton, A. (1989) *Invitation to Self Management*. Ruislip: Dab Hand Press.

Stevenson, J. and Cook, C. (1977) *The Slump: Society and Politics during the Depression*. London: Cape.

Stoecker, R. (2013) *Research Methods for Community Change: A Project-Based Approach*, 2nd edn. London: Sage.

Syrett, S. and North. D. (2010) Between economic competiveness and social inclusion: New Labour and the economic revival of deprived neighbourhoods, *Local Economy*, 25(5–6): 476–93.

Tasker, L. (1980) Practice and theory in community work: a case for reconciliation, in P. Henderson, D. Jones and D. N. Thomas (eds) *The Boundaries of Change in Community Work*. London: Allen & Unwin.

Taylor, A. J. P. (1965) *English History, 1914–1945*. Oxford: Oxford University Press.

Taylor, M. (1979) Managing community resources, *Talking Point*, no. 13. London: Association of Community Workers.

Taylor, M. (1992) *Signposts to Community Development*. London: Community Development Foundation and the National Coalition of Neighbourhoods.

Taylor, M. and Presley, F. (1987) *Community Work in the UK 1982–6* (ed. G. Chanan). London: Library Association Publishing in association with Calouste Gulbenkian Foundation.

Tett, L. (2006) *Community Education, Lifelong Learning and Social Inclusion*, 2nd edn. Edinburgh: Dunedin Academic Press.

Thane, P. (1989) *Foundations of the Welfare State*. London: Longman.

Thomas, D. N. (1983) *The Making of Community Work*. London: George Allen & Unwin.

Thompson, E. P. (1977) *William Morris: From Romantic to Revolutionary*. London: Merlin.

Thorns, D. C. (1976) *The Quest for Community: Social Aspects of Residential Growth*. London: George Allen & Unwin.

Tilly, C. (2004) *Social Movements, 1768–2004*. Boulder, CO: Paradigm Publishers.

Tönnies, F. (1955) *Community and Association*. London: Routledge & Kegan Paul.

Townsend, P. (1962) *The Last Refuge: A Survey of Residential Institutions and Homes for the Aged in England and Wales*. London: Routledge & Kegan Paul.

Toynbee, P. (2013) We must all share the blame for our "useless" politicians, *Guardian*. 31 December.

Trevithick, P. (2012) *Social Work Skills and Knowledge: A Practice Handbook*, 3rd edn. Maidenhead: Open University Press/McGraw-Hill Education.

Turbett, C. (2014) *Doing Radical Social Work*. Basingstoke: Palgrave Macmillan.

Twelvetrees (1983) Whither community work? in D.N. Thomas (ed.) *Community Work in the Eighties*. London: National Institute for Social Work.

Twelvetrees, A. (2008) *Community Work*, 4th edn. Basingstoke: Palgrave Macmillan.

Unemployment Unit and Youth Aid (1993) *Working Brief*, February/March. London: Unemployment Unit and Youth Aid.

United Nations (1959) *European Seminar on Community Development and Social Welfare in Urban Areas*. Geneva: United Nations.

Waddington, P. (1983) Looking ahead: community work into the 1980s, in D. N. Thomas (ed.) *Community Work in the Eighties*. London: National Institute for Social Work.

Wagner, G. (1988) *Residential Care: A Positive Choice*. London: National Institute for Social Work/HMSO.

Walby, S. (2011) *The Future of Feminism*. Cambridge: Polity.

Walker, A. (1987) Introduction: a policy for two nations, in A. Walker and C. Walker (eds) *The Growing Divide: A Social Audit 1979–1987*. London: Child Poverty Action Group.

Ware, V. (1991) *Beyond the Pale: White Women, Racism and History*. London: Verso.

Webb, S. A. (2009) Against difference and diversity in social work: the case of human rights, *International Journal of Social Welfare*, 18(2): 307–16.

Webb, S. A. (2011) Nothing in common? Guerrilla ontologies in rethinking 'community' and community engagement. Unpublished paper, University of Newcastle, Australia.

Weber, M. (1930) *The Protestant Ethic and the Spirit of Capitalism* (first published in German in 1904–5). London: Allen & Unwin.

Weber, M. (1978) *Economy and Society: An Outline of Interpretive Sociology* (2 vols). Berkeley: University of California Press.

Weston, C. (1993) Firms to receive subsidy on jobs, *Guardian*, 17 March.

Whitting, G., Burton, P., Means, R. and Stewart, M. (1986) *The Urban Programme and the Young Unemployed*. Inner Cities Research Programme. London: Department of the Environment.

Wilkinson, R. and Pickett, K. (2010) *The Spirit Level: Why Equality Is Better for Everyone*. London: Penguin.

Williams, F. (1991) *Social Policy: A Critical Introduction*. Cambridge: Polity.

Williams, R. (1976) *Keywords*. London: Fontana/Croom Helm.

Williams, R. (2011) The government need to know how afraid people are, *New Statesman*, 9 June.

Williamson, H. (1988) Youth workers, the MSC and the Youth Training Scheme, in T. Jeffs and M. Smith (eds) *Welfare and Youth Work Practice*. Basingstoke: Macmillan Education.

Wilmott, P. (1963) *The Evolution of a Community*. London: Routledge & Kegan Paul.

Wilmott, P. (1989) *Community Initiatives: Patterns and Prospects*. London: Policy Studies Institute.

Wilmott, P. and Thomas, D. (1984) *Community in Social Policy*. London: Policy Studies Institute.

Wilson, E. (1977) *Women and the Welfare State*. London: Tavistock.

Wood, J. and Cracknell, R. (2013) *Ethnic Minorities in Politics, Government and Public Life*. Standard Note SN/SG/1156. London: House of Commons Library.

Woodin, M. and Lucas, C. (2004) *Green Alternatives to Globalisation: A Manifesto*. London: Pluto Press.

Worley, C. (2005) 'It's not about race. It's about the community': New Labour and 'community cohesion', *Critical Social Policy*, 25: 483–96.

Younghusband, E. L. (1959) *Report of the Working Party on Social Workers in the Local Authority Health and Welfare Services*. London: HMSO.

Appendix   Select Community Development Project bibliography

Benwell CDP (1978) *Slums on the Drawing Board, Final Report No. 4*. Newcastle: Benwell CDP.

Birmingham CDP (1978) *Leasehold Loopholes, Final Report No. 5*. Birmingham and Oxford: Birmingham CDP Research Team and the Social Evaluation Unit, Oxford University.

Birmingham CDP (1987) *Youth on the Dole, Final Report No. 4*. Birmingham and Oxford: Birmingham CDP Research Team and the Social Evaluation Unit, Oxford University.

Butterworth, E., Lees, R. and Arnold, P. (1980) *The Challenge of Community Work, Final Report of Batley CDP*, Papers in Community Studies, No. 24. York: University of York.

Canning Town CDP (1976) *Growth and Decline: Canning Town's Economy, 1846–1946*. London: Canning Town CDP.

Canning Town CDP (1978a) *Canning Town to North Woolwich: The Aims of Industry?* London: Canning Town CDP.

Canning Town CDP (1978b) *Canning Town's Declining Community Income*. London: Canning Town CDP.

CDP (1977a) *Gilding the Ghetto: The State and the Poverty Experiments*. London: Community Development Project Inter-project Editorial Team.

COP (1977b) *The Costs of Industrial Change*. London: Community Development Project and Inter-project Editorial Team.

CDP IIU (1975) *The Poverty of the Improvement Programme*. London: CDP Information and Intelligence Unit.

CDP IIU (1976a) *Profits against Houses*. London: COP Information and Intelligence Unit.

COP IIU (1976b) *Whatever Happened to Council Housing?* London: CDP Information and Intelligence Unit.

Analysing community work

CDP PEC (1979) *The State and the Local Economy*. London: CDP PEC and Publications Distributive Co-operative.

CIS/CDP (1976) *Cutting the Welfare State (Who Profits?)* London: Counter Information Services and CDP.

Corina, L. (1977) *Oldham CDP: An Assessment of its Impact and Influence on the Local Authority*, Papers in Community Studies, No. 9. York: University of York.

Corina, L., Collis, P. and Crosby, C. (1979) *Oldham CDP: The Final Report*. York: University of York.

Coventry CDP (1978a) *Coventry and Hillfields: Prosperity and the Persistence of Inequality, Final Report, Part 1*. Coventry: Coventry CDP.

Coventry CDP (1978b) *Background Working Papers, Final Report, Part 2*. Coventry: Coventry CDP.

North Tyneside CDP (1978a) *North Shields: Working Class Politics and Housing 1900–77, Final Report*, Vol. 1. Newcastle: Newcastle upon Tyne Polytechnic.

North Tyneside CDP (1978b) *North Shields: Organizing for Change in a Working Class Area, Final Report*, Vol. 3. Newcastle: Newcastle upon Tyne Polytechnic.

North Tyneside CDP (1978c) *North Shields: Organizing for Change in a Working Class Area: The Action Groups, Final Report*, Vol. 4. Newcastle: Newcastle upon Tyne Polytechnic.

North Tyneside CDP (1978d) *Women's Work, Final Report*, Vol. 5. Newcastle: Newcastle upon Tyne Polytechnic.

North Tyneside CDP (1978e) *In and Out of Work: A Study of Unemployment, Low Pay and Income Maintenance Services*. Newcastle: Newcastle upon Tyne Polytechnic.

Penn, R. and Alden, J. (1977) *Upper Afan CDP Final Report to Sponsors: Joint Report by Action Team and Research Team Directors, Cardiff, University of Wales, Institute of Science and Technology*. Cardiff: University of Wales.

Index

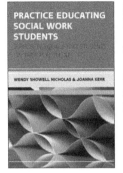

Practice Educating Social Work Students
Supporting qualifying students on their placements

Wendy Showell Nicholas and Joanna Kerr

ISBN: 978-0-335-26282-3 (Paperback)
eBook: 978-0-335-26283-0
2015

This brand new book is essential reading for anyone involved in practice educating social work students. Whether you are an on-site or off-site practice educator, or a workplace supervisor, the book will guide you through your role, providing practical and straightforward advice about the process from start to finish.

Key features include:

- Guidence on how to assess and support students to achieve the very best
- Explores how to tackle difficult conversations and create action plans
- Contains many practical tips, handy checklists and realistic examples

www.openup.co.uk

OPEN UNIVERSITY PRESS
McGraw - Hill Education

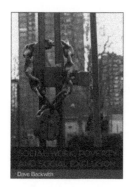

Social Work, Poverty and Social Inclusion

Dave Backwith

ISBN: 978-0-335-24585-7 (Paperback)
eBook: 978-0-335-24586-4
2015

This book relates poverty and social exclusion to social work practice, offering a fresh approach to the challenges social workers face in helping clients out of poverty. *Social Work, Poverty and Social Inclusion* supports students in developing relationship-based and community-oriented approaches that can actively alleviate poverty.

Key features include:

- Numerous quotations and vignettes
- "What Do You Think?" exercises
- Explores the relation of poverty and social exclusion

www.openup.co.uk

OPEN UNIVERSITY PRESS
McGraw - Hill Education

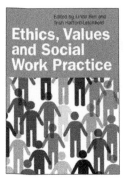

Ethics, Values and Social Work Practice

Linda Bell and Hafford-Letchfield

ISBN: 978-0-335-24529-I (Paperback)
eBook: 978-0-335-24530-7

2015

Ethics, Values and Social Work Practice is a brand new text offering students and social work practitioners a contemporary and relevant introduction to the central role of ethics and values in their work. This book offers a fresh perspective on ethics and values in the context of everyday social work practice, and provides an accessible route into the key theories, as well as useful strategies, tips and tools for practice.

Key features include:

- Discussion points for individual reflection or ethical debates
- Case studies based on likely scenarios from practice
- Chapter summaries and key points for social work practice

www.openup.co.uk

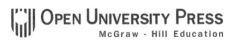 OPEN UNIVERSITY PRESS
McGraw - Hill Education

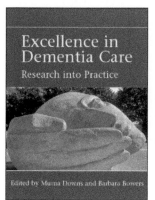

EXCELLENCE IN DEMENTIA CARE: RESEARCH INTO PRACTICE

Murna Downs and Barbara Bowers

9780335223756 (Paperback)
2008

eBook also available

"Written by leading theorists from a range of countries, this comprehensive text is a unique achievement. Despite there being 46 contributors, there is a consistent voice addressing current thinking in dementia care, with good cross referencing. Expertise of researchers, practitioners and academic tutors is brought together in a stimulating, informative and sometimes provocative read."
Nursing Standard

In addressing the many complex issues related to offering support to people with dementia and those who care for them, this timely textbook is unique in emphasising strategies for creating sustainable change in practice.

The book includes examples from a range of countries, drawn from research, practice wisdom and, most importantly, from the experience of people with dementia and their families.

Offers valuable insights on how to:
- Provide competent and compassionate care for people with Alzheimer's Disease and other dementias
- Build systems to provide effective care
- Encourage collaboration among multi disciplinary professionals and users and carers

www.openup.co.uk

OPEN UNIVERSITY PRESS
McGraw - Hill Education